TEACHING YOGA
ADJUSTING ASANA

MELANIE COOPER

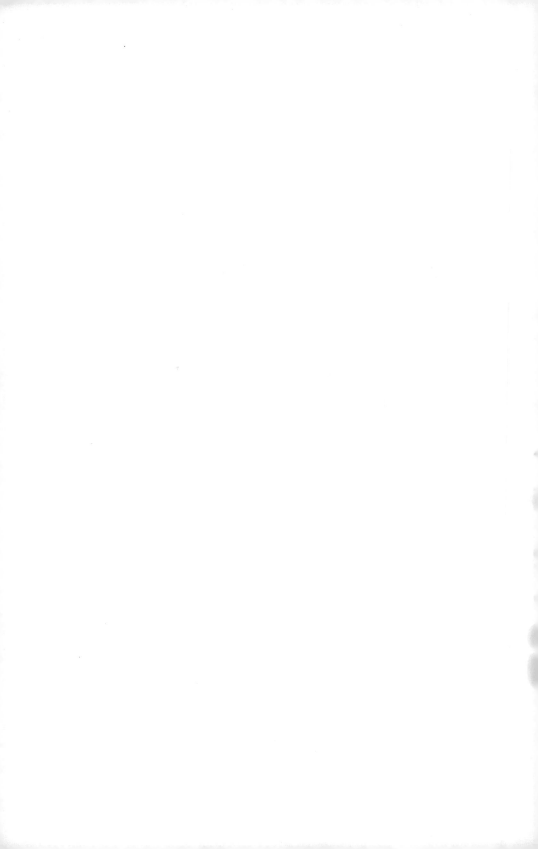

TEACHING YOGA
ADJUSTING ASANA

BASED ON THE ASHTANGA PRIMARY SERIES
A HANDBOOK FOR STUDENTS AND TEACHERS

MELANIE COOPER

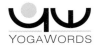

YOGAWORDS

The author and publisher disclaim, as far as the law allows, any liability arising directly or indirectly from the use, or misuse, of the information contained in this book.

Teaching Yoga, Adjusting Asana
Based on the Ashtanga Primary Series
A handbook for students and teachers

First published in 2013 by YogaWords Ltd

ISBN 978-1906756-20-8

Models: Melanie Cooper and Emil Lime
Managing editor: Zoë Blanc
Editor: James Hodgson
Design: Boguś Machnik / Spiral Path Design
Jacket photography: Yard Studio / www.yardphoto.co.uk

A catalogue record for this book is available from the British Library

Printed and bound in the UK by Martins the Printers, Berwick-upon-Tweed

This book has been printed on paper that is sourced and harvested from sustainable forests and is FSC accredited

YogaWords Ltd
32 Clarendon Road
London N8 0DJ

www.yogawords.com

CONTENTS

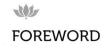

FOREWORD

I first started practising Ashtanga yoga in 1993. Pretty much from my first class I was hooked. I had always been active – with swimming, cycling, circuit training and, I am not too embarrassed to admit, aerobics. But when I discovered Ashtanga I knew I had found my thing. I loved (and still love) to challenge myself physically – with Ashtanga I could do that and afterwards, instead of feeling hyper, I would feel like I was floating – on cloud nine.

I soon realised that the benefits of Ashtanga were huge. The feeling of well-being started to stay with me and physically I was in better shape than I had ever been – even now I'm in my mid-forties, I continue to get stronger, more flexible and able to do things I could never dream of in my twenties. Mentally, I came out of my daydream and started to engage more fully with reality. I started to see my patterns of behaviour, and the chattering voice inside my head grew quieter and stiller. At around the time I started to practise yoga, I developed chronic fatigue syndrome. My yoga practice really kept me going, physically and mentally. Yoga became a huge part of my life. I also started to become interested in yoga philosophy and found a lot that I could apply to my life to help me live more honestly and authentically.

In those days yoga was far less popular than it is now. The usual assumption if you practised yoga was that you sat around knitting cardigans, eating lentils and chanting 'om'. 'No,' I would explain, 'I do Ashtanga – that's different,' but no one really understood.

In 1997 I took voluntary redundancy from my job as a librarian, intending to become a massage therapist. Then a friend who was a yoga teacher asked me to teach his class when he went on holiday. I said 'no way' and he said 'yes way' and to cut a long story short I taught his class and absolutely loved it. He then gave me a permanent class and I was offered more classes. Before I knew it, I had become a yoga teacher. I have been teaching at health clubs, yoga centres and for various other organisations ever since.

In 2003 I went for the first time to Mysore to study with Sri K. Pattabhi Jois. In 2004 I started to assist Hamish Hendry, the most senior Ashtanga teacher in the UK. Also in 2004 I did the Ashtanga teacher-training at Brahmani Yoga in India. They invited me back there to teach and I have been teaching in Goa every winter ever since. From 2006 I have been a senior teacher on the Yoga Alliance teacher-training courses run there. And since 2008 I have co-taught a Yoga Alliance-accredited intensive course at Bristol City Yoga. From 2011 I have led the morning Mysore self-practice at the Life Centre, Islington. For over 15 years I have taught general gym classes, counted led primaries, beginners courses, advanced workshops and adjustment workshops for teachers. I have worked in upmarket health clubs, beach resorts and local authority gyms, as well as at holiday camps, hippie and punk festivals. I have taught people with mental health problems, primary school teachers, teenagers, children, OAPs and loved it all.

This book came about after I put together a manual (with some pho-tos and a brief description of how to do the adjustments) for a workshop I was teaching. I was amazed at how quickly and accurately people picked up the adjustments with the help of what I had written. Then I wrote notes on teaching for the Bristol intensive course. The feedback I got for the notes and photos was overwhelmingly positive and I started to think, *this looks like a book*, and the project has grown from there.

I have always loved teaching yoga. As I have developed as a teacher, I have started to love teaching other people to become teachers – at this stage in my career that is what most interests and inspires me. This book has come about from my desire to share knowledge about the practice I love – yoga – and in particular Ashtanga yoga.

ACKNOWLEDGEMENTS

This book is really a group effort. I could not have done it without a huge amount of help and inspiration from so many people over the years.

Thanks go to my teachers: Oz, Hamish Hendry and Julie Martin – you rock.

Thanks to everyone at Ashtanga Yoga London – my yoga family.

Thanks to all at Brahmani – I have learned so much and had so much fun.

Thanks to all my students over the years, but Fitness First Tottenham you have a special place in my heart.

Thanks to my friends, especially the ones who read the manuscript and gave help and advice – Norman Blair, Inna Cos, Adriane Klumpp, Diane Gabrysiak, Georgina Evans, Ruth Westoby and a huge, huge thank you to Yonnie Fung.

Thanks to Laura Gilmore for her initial encouragement.

Thanks to Chun Lee for doing the layout and making it look like a book.

Thanks to Oliver Fokerd for the photos and the beautiful Satsanga retreat for the location.

Thanks to Mark Singleton for his help, especially in Chapters 6 and 10.

Thanks to Bryony Bird for the referencing.

Thanks to Rocco Marinelli for the editing.

Thanks to Amy Willesee for the read-through and encouragement.

Thanks to Zoë Blanc at YogaWords, and to James Hodgson for copy-editing.

And thanks to Emil Lime – my model and husband – for all his love and support.

Special mention to Brahmani Yoga and Bristol City Yoga for the excellent teacher-training programmes – this book really owes everything to them.

And thanks to the publishers, YogaWords, for believing in the project.

INTRODUCTION

This book is primarily about teaching yoga and contains much information that will be of interest and use to teachers and students of all styles of yoga. I am an Ashtanga teacher and so the book is based on the Ashtanga Primary Series.

Before I go any further I want to state clearly that this book is not about Ashtanga yoga as it is traditionally taught in Mysore, and I am not trying to give the 'correct Mysore point of view'. I have the utmost respect for Pattabhi Jois and Sharath and their teaching methods. I was taught myself mainly by a teacher who remains very faithful to the traditional style and I am very grateful and consider myself very lucky to have been taught this way. I have also studied in Mysore with Pattabhi Jois and Sharath and completely loved the experience and gained a huge amount from it, but I do not pretend to speak for them and they have not endorsed this book.

I think that there is no doubt about the authenticity and integrity of Pattabhi Jois and Sharath. Their teaching method has produced some of the most accomplished, knowledgeable and sincere yoga practitioners around today, but the reality facing most new yoga teachers is that most of their classes are in gyms where it is not possible to teach in the Mysore style. Most of these classes are only one hour long and are open to all levels. Most of the students are practising only once or twice a week. In this situation a new way of teaching Ashtanga has emerged – a general led class – and this is what *Teaching Yoga, Adjusting Asana* is about. But it is my hope that this book will be useful to many different categories of yoga practitioner.

So, firstly this book is for newly qualified teachers teaching in gyms. I have been there myself and I know the frustrations and joys of teaching in this way. It is not an easy path – it can be immensely rewarding but also hugely frustrating. The fact that yoga in gyms has thrived for nearly two decades is testament to the huge benefits yoga has to offer, and the dedication and hard work of all the gym-based yoga teachers. We have seen many fads and fashions come and go in the gyms over the years and many attempts by the gyms to outdo us in our own territory, but yoga classes remain perennially popular. I hope this book will give you support, ideas and food for thought.

This book is also for teachers of all kinds of yoga. It is a source of sadness to me that some yoga teachers look more for the divisions between types of yoga rather than what we have in common. I feel we are all doing essentially the same thing but with different emphases to cater for all the different personalities and body types doing asana:

- We all do asana, pranayama, bandhas and dristi.
- We all have to deal with students and their injuries.
- We all have to work out how to communicate effectively.
- We all try to explain the spiritual aspects of yoga.
- We all have to deal with the same ethical difficulties and dilemmas.
- The chapter on deepening the Primary Series gives ideas for workshops that would work for many styles of yoga.
- The adjustment chapter is applicable to all who would like to start working in a more hands-on way with their students.

I hope there is much in this book that will help and inspire teachers of many forms of yoga.

I also hope that students of yoga will find much of help and interest here. The in-depth information about the breathing, bandhas and dristi could help students of any level deepen their practice and their understanding of yoga in general. This applies especially to more advanced students who are thinking of starting to teach and those already on teacher-training courses.

The feedback I have received from people who have read this book during the editorial process has been very positive. The book has been tried out by both newly qualified and more experienced yoga teachers, and by beginner and more experienced students. All of them found information and ideas that were helpful and interesting and useful to them in their practice and teaching.

The book is basically in two parts: Chapters 1 to 7, which focus on the process of teaching as a whole; and Chapters 8 to 11, which are primarily practical and relate to the individual asana. Chapter 1 gives general information about various important aspects of teaching. Chapters 2, 3 and 4 cover the breath, bandhas and dristi. For each of these you will find basic information about technique, contraindications and benefits, as well as ideas about how to teach it. Where relevant, the information is divided into scientific aspects and more yogic aspects and wherever possible I have included references to scientific studies or yogic texts. Chapter 5 covers injuries – how they are caused, how to prevent them and how to work with students who are injured. In Chapter 6 I give some ideas about how to teach the spiritual aspects of yoga and Chapter 7 explores the ethics of yoga teaching through the structure of the yamas and niyamas. Chapter 8 deals with teaching points: what to say, how to say it and ideas for phrases for each asana in the Primary Series. In Chapter 9 the whole Primary Series is given with the Sanskrit count. This gives the breath and movements into and out of each pose. In Chapter 10 I give various stretches and strengthening exercises that can help students to work on the Primary Series and ideas for how to put these together for workshop-style classes. The final chapter of the book deals with adjustments. First I give some background about why we adjust, how adjustments work and how as teachers we can make it as safe as possible. Then for each posture, I have included photographs of the adjustment and succinct clear instructions of how to carry out the adjustment.

As a teacher, it is a good idea sometimes to choose a focus for a class. For example, if you have noticed that your students do not seem to be breathing properly, you could teach a whole class focused on the breath. Read the relevant chapter on breathing. Look for three pieces of information to emphasise during the class (if you try to give too much information, people tend to go into brain overload and switch off). Maybe choose one scientific way in which the special breathing can benefit the body, one of the yogic ways in which breathing affects the body and one of the breathing exercises. Take some time in the class to talk about the breath in more depth, explain clearly how to do it, why we do it and what the benefits are. I find if students know why they are doing something, and understand the theory behind it, they are more likely to carry on doing it.

If you feel you are always saying the same things and worry that you are lacking in inspiration, look at the teaching points. These are given in the chapters on breath and bandhas, as well as in Chapter 8, which is devoted exclusively to teaching points. Do not necessarily take my points and copy them, although this could be a good way to start, but use them for sparking ideas and themes in a class. For example, you could teach a whole class focused on the foundation and the use of the hands and feet (see Chapter 8).

If you want to learn more hands-on adjustment work, get together with two yoga friends. One of you will be reading out instructions, one will be the student and the third will be doing the adjustment. Try two or three asana in a session and follow the instructions given in Chapter 11. Experiment with different levels of pressure and what feels good. Then try the adjustment on a student you know well, and build up slowly from there.

All this is in no way meant to replace a teacher-training course or study with a senior teacher. It is intended as a supplement to give you ideas and inspiration and to help you find your voice as a teacher. I taught for seven years before going on a course. I made it up as I went along and learned by my mistakes. My classes were busy and popular and no one died, but my teaching definitely improved a huge amount after I went on my teacher-training course – I highly, highly recommend it.

My intention in writing this book is to share and pass on information and ideas I have gathered in nearly two decades of practising and teaching. I learned from my teachers and students and I have a huge desire to share this learning. I find the process of teaching very satisfying and in teaching I learn myself.

TEACHING YOGA

Teaching is an ongoing process. In the beginning you teach what you know. As time goes on, your understanding deepens, your knowledge expands and your teaching develops. Your practice is a major resource for your teaching. As you go along, your practice will help your teaching and in turn your teaching will help your practice.

In this chapter, we will consider certain basic issues involved in teaching yoga, such as how you communicate both verbally and physically, how you present yourself, and how you deal with common problems associated with learners of all levels of experience.

BEFORE YOU START

MYSORE STYLE

The legend states that Sri K. Pattabhi Jois (Guruji) and his teacher Sri Krishnamacharya together translated an ancient text called the *Yoga Korunta*. From that they refined a system of asana (yoga poses) called Ashtanga Yoga. Guruji taught this system in Mysore from the late 1930s until his death in 2009. 'Mysore style' has come to mean the way in which Guruji (and now his grandson Sharath) taught yoga. Guruji and Sharath taught 'self-practice style', whereby each student is initially shown a small portion of the sequence, which they become comfortable with before being given the next posture, and so on, until they build up the whole sequence.

Mysore style requires great discipline and regular practice from the student, so it is difficult to teach in this way if you are working at a gym where students tend to be transient or irregular. Most gym classes are 'led classes' in which the teacher talks through the sequence and students follow along.

If you are an Ashtanga yoga teacher, I would strongly recommend you go to Mysore to study if at all possible.

HOW TO PRESENT YOURSELF

As a yoga teacher, you are the leader of your class. This means not only setting an agenda of postures to be taught, but also setting a certain tone, which can be just as important in creating a positive, purposeful learning environment. Use your personal appearance to project the kind of atmosphere that you want to achieve.

- Have a wash (including your feet).
- Wear clean clothes.
- Choose clothes that are neat, that do not distract and that show your body so that people can see clearly what you are doing.
- Tie your hair back so it does not trail on students.
- Do not wear jewellery that is likely to cut someone or trail on students during an adjustment.
- Cut your fingernails and toenails.
- Start and finish your classes on time.

WAYS OF LEARNING

There are three main tools you can use to guide your students into an asana:

- explanation
- demonstration
- physical adjustment

The Mysore-style method of teaching yoga consists of using minimal verbal explanation, and teaching as much as you can with your hands. The reasoning is that verbal communication will break the flow of the practice and take someone out of the body and into the mind. For some people, an explanation alongside an adjustment will be very helpful. It is good to use a mixture of the three methods when teaching a led class. Sometimes it is appropriate to tell the student what you mean, sometimes to show them by demonstrating and sometimes to physically put them in a posture with your hands.

If you are teaching a general led class in a gym, then you will use a mixture of all three approaches, but, particularly in large classes, explanation and demonstration will be more important and physical adjustment less so.

EXPLANATION

How you communicate is just as important as *what* you communicate. Teaching in a genuine way is the key to being a great teacher. If it's clear that you are speaking from experience, you'll win your students' confidence and trust.

Initially as yoga teachers, we learn what to say and repeat what our teachers have told us, but later on, when we have all the information firmly in our head, we start to communicate from the heart (see Chapter 8, Teaching Points). Step outside of yourself and make a conscious effort to consider how your students will process your words, bearing in mind the following:

Patience: It is important to be patient and gentle, especially with beginners. Try to remember how you felt when you were a beginner yourself. Beginners should be allowed to go at their own pace and build up their practice slowly. Make sure you do not over-correct a beginner. Let them make mistakes; if everything they do is being corrected, they will leave feeling they got everything wrong.

Body awareness: Some people have very little connection with their body. When you say something like 'draw the shoulders down', they may have no idea what you mean. Watch for these kinds of misunderstanding and find another way to communicate your meaning.

Emotional holding: Some people have patterns of holding their body that are related to emotional issues. A common example is hunching up the shoulders for protection. You can encourage them to relax their shoulders, but if they are not ready to deal with the feeling of vulnerability or lack of protection, they will not do it.

Clarity and simplicity: Say less not more. If you say too much, either by making your explanations too wordy or by giving too many teaching points, the students are likely either to become confused or to stop listening, or both. It is best to stick to a few clear and concise points, so the students learn a few things really well. For beginners, keep repeating the same words, especially when you are referring to the breath and bandhas. The instructions then become an internal script that will always stay with them. If a student cannot understand what you are saying, it is your responsibility as a teacher to find a way of helping them to understand.

Using you own practice as a resource for your teaching: When you are in a posture, notice what you do. For example, notice which muscles are engaged, which are relaxed and where the stretch happens. When teaching in a general class however, make sure that you give instructions that apply to a range of different body types. Some instructions can be applied generally, but some are specific to certain body types. Avoid limiting your instructions to those that only suit your own body.

Knowing your limits: Because you are a teacher, some people will assume that you have super-human knowledge of everything under the sun. Clearly none of us does. You are just a yoga teacher; when you are asked questions to which you do not know the answer, it is important not to get drawn in. Always be honest and respond with a simple 'I don't know'.

DEMONSTRATION

When teaching, how you demonstrate the postures is important. Consider how best to make your demonstration seen and understood by your students.

Protect yourself: When demonstrating, the first thing to remember is to be careful with your own body. If you are continually demonstrating when you are not warmed up, only demonstrating on one side, or not breathing properly, then you are going to hurt yourself sooner or later. Be gentle with yourself.

Modification: When demonstrating to beginners, do not do your full version of the posture. While it might inspire some people, it will make others feel they cannot do it and will never be able to do it (which in many cases is true). Always explain different options; start with the easiest and then show how the posture can develop as students improve their flexibility and strength. Then, as the class joins in, go back and demonstrate the easiest option yourself.

Where to stand: Make sure students have a clear view of you when you demonstrate. There is no point in demonstrating something at the front of the class if everyone has got their back to you. Think about where students will best be able to see you.

Mirroring: When demonstrating, it is best to mirror. 'Mirroring' means demonstrating a pose in such a way that allows a student to see their own mirror image when they look at you. This can get confusing for you because you will be doing something with your left, but saying you are doing it with your right. Wherever possible, avoid using verbal cues such as 'right' and 'left'. Instead, use 'bent leg' or 'front leg' or wave your arm and say 'this arm'. Not only does this avoid your own confusion, but it will help the students as well.

ADJUSTMENT

There are three levels of adjustment: 'correction', where you use your hands gently to correct a posture; 'guidance', where you gently show the direction a student should take in the posture; and full 'adjustment', where you take an experienced student deeper into the posture.

Beginners: When teaching beginners, it is important to be gentle and to use corrections rather than adjustments. These corrections help a student find their alignment, their foundation, relax their shoulders or connect to their core strength.

Intermediate students: With intermediate-level students, you can use guidance: show the way in a posture without pushing them deeper.

Experienced students: When a student is more experienced, and if their alignment and breathing are good, it can be helpful to give a stronger but always sensitive adjustment. (See Chapter 11, Adjustments.)

SAFETY FIRST

You will come across a wide variety of students, some of whom will have particular health issues that may affect their yoga practice. Considering the following points will help you to avoid problems, but it is also a really good idea to do a first aid certificate course before you begin teaching so that you know what to do if something does go wrong.

EXISTING INJURIES AND HEALTH CONDITIONS

If someone has an acute (very recent) painful injury, they should not practise yoga. A very recent injury (within the previous 48 hours) should be rested, iced, compressed and elevated. An older injury can be worked around: make sure the student does not do anything that causes pain, especially a sharp or 'electrical' pain. (See Chapter 5, Injuries.)

There are also long-term health conditions that can affect a person's ability to practise yoga. The following is not an exhaustive list, just some ideas of the kind of health issues that may make a general yoga class inadvisable.

- heart condition: check with GP
- high blood pressure: check with GP and do not do any inversions
- recent surgery: check with GP
- herniated disk

When in doubt, ask the student to check with their GP before they partic-ipate in a yoga class. If you do not feel you can work with a student in your class, you can always refer them to a yoga therapy or remedial yoga class.

PAIN

Pain is a problematic issue for a yoga teacher. People experience many sensations in the body when they practise yoga. Some sensations are connected with safe stretching of muscles, while other sensations signal imminent damage. You need to help your students recognise the difference. While you can offer some guidance in distinguishing safe sensations from dangerous sensations, ultimately you need to give the student the responsibility of listening to their own body.

Many people will start with some idea of having to 'go through the pain barrier' – the 'no pain no gain' mentality. This attitude should be strongly discouraged. Painful sensations in the joints must not be tolerated, particularly when it is sharp pain. Pain in a joint means that the tendons or ligaments or cartilage are being stressed. This is especially the case when the pain occurs in the spine or the knees. A dull ache in the middle of a muscle normally indicates safe stretching of a muscle.

As a teacher, err on the side of caution. Suggest the student go to the edge of the pain-free zone, however far that is, then relax and breathe there. This approach is especially important if the area has already been injured.

There is a balance to be struck between pushing too hard and maybe causing injury, and doing nothing and getting nowhere. This is the important yogic idea of allowing the stretch to happen: somewhere between passive and active. (See Chapter 5, Injuries.)

PREGNANCY

Yoga can be highly beneficial during pregnancy, helping to relieve discomfort and pain, and preparing the body and mind for childbirth and parenthood. However, there are certain safety guidelines to bear in mind.

New students: When someone has never done yoga before and thinks she should start because she is pregnant, Ashtanga yoga is definitely not the right place for her to start. Direct her to a 'yoga for pregnancy' class.

The Mysore guideline: The Mysore guideline is not to practise for the first three months of pregnancy, as this is the most vulnerable time, especially around the fourth, eighth and twelfth weeks. After resting for the first three months, the student can practise with modifications.

Relaxin: This is a hormone produced during pregnancy to enable the body to open for the baby to be born. At some point in pregnancy (exactly when varies from woman to woman), relaxin is released and the body becomes a lot more flexible. It is important that the pregnant student does not go to her maximum in postures, as her ligaments and tendons can be permanently stretched and her joints destabilised. Relaxin can still be in the body after the birth and during breast-feeding, so care should also be taken post-natally.

Modification: If an existing Ashtanga yoga student wishes to carry on doing Ashtanga yoga during her pregnancy, she will need to modify many of the postures to make them safe and comfortable.

I would suggest that if you want to teach yoga to pregnant women, you attend a 'yoga for pregnancy' course to learn how to conduct a class safely.

PERIODS

The Mysore view is that you should not practise for the first three days of your period. After the first three days, you can practise but leave out inversions and use bandhas very gently. This is a fairly contentious issue. Some people will argue that banning women from practising while they are menstruating is old-fashioned and unnecessary. Some women feel better when they practise during their period, some feel worse.

I would suggest that you tell students the Mysore guidelines, but also advise students to notice how they feel. If practising while on her period makes a student feel drained and tired or makes her cramps worse, then obviously she should take a rest from yoga during this time. If it relieves her pain and makes her feel better, then maybe she should practise gently, with no inversions and only gentle bandhas.

MENTAL HEALTH, ADDICTION AND EATING DISORDERS

If a student has serious mental health issues, it is best not to let them practise in a general class. Direct them to a class specifically for people with mental health problems, where the teacher and students will have proper support.

Ashtanga yoga often attracts people with addictive personalities. Some students practising Ashtanga either have current issues or have had issues with drugs or eating disorders. As a yoga teacher, it is not your role to get involved with helping people directly with these issues. However, you do need to know that if a student is anorexic and extremely thin, their bones can be brittle and you should be extremely cautious about giving them adjustments. If a student tries to attend a class and is evidently under the influence of drugs or alcohol, you should not let them practise.

INSURANCE

Make sure you have adequate insurance, which should include public liability, malpractice and professional indemnity policies. Public liability insurance protects you against any claims from students or other members of the public who have injured themselves due to environmental causes, such as faulty equipment in your yoga studio – for example, tripping on a loose tile in the changing room. Malpractice insurance protects you against claims from students who say they have injured themselves doing asana in your class. Professional indemnity insurance protects you against claims from students who have lost out on earnings due to injuries they sustained in your class. There are other optional forms of insurance you can add on, such as help with legal or accountancy fees resulting from a tax office investigation or claims arising from any products you might use. While it is not actually illegal to teach without insurance, most gyms and yoga centres do require it. If you do not have insurance and something does go wrong, you can end up with a huge bill for legal costs and damages. You also have a moral responsibility to make sure that your students are protected in case of injuries or accidents. Insurance is relatively inexpensive and easy to arrange. Check whether the governing body overseeing your teacher-training course offers a group discount policy.

BEGINNERS

Students who are new to yoga will need particularly careful handling. To help them prepare for their first class, you might give them a sheet of general guidelines (see box opposite). These will help them to avoid the following problems commonly experienced by first-time students.

Feeling dizzy: This could be due to low blood pressure or low blood sugar. For low blood pressure suggest they:

- eat something salty thirty minutes before class (salty food raises blood pressure)
- do only very gentle ujjayi breathing (see page 29) – strong ujjayi breath may lower the blood pressure too much
- take extra time coming up and out of standing forward bends

If dizzy feelings are very strong and persistent, you could suggest that the student check with their GP.

Students with low blood-sugar levels should eat a complex carbohydrate snack 30 minutes before class. This will give a sustained release of energy throughout the class and avoid blood-sugar levels going too low.

Feeling nauseous: This can be due to toxins releasing into the blood stream and should stop happening in time. Suggest they drink more water generally, as drinking water helps to flush toxins from the system.

Wanting to drink water: It is best not to drink while practising asana. Firstly, it feels uncomfortable to have water in the stomach when practising. Secondly, in yogic terms during an asana practice we are trying to build up internal heat – drinking water counteracts this. However, to avoid being too harsh, if a beginner really feels like they need to drink, suggest they take little sips.

Struggling to keep up: If a student is struggling to keep up physically, allow them to rest. During the sun salutations, replace downward dog with child pose; during the standing postures, they can rest in Tadasana, and during the sitting postures in Sukasana.

GENERAL GUIDELINES FOR BEGINNERS

- Yoga is best done on an empty stomach, so do not eat just before class and leave two hours after a full meal and one hour after a light snack.
- Do not drink for 30 minutes before a yoga class.
- Wash before class.
- Wear clean, comfortable clothing that will not restrict your movement.
- Let your teacher know if you have injuries or health issues.
- Wash your mat regularly.
- When you are on your period, either rest completely or do a very gentle yoga practice.
- If you are pregnant, let your teacher know straight away.

SUMMARY

In this chapter we have explored some of the principles of successful yoga teaching. However, perhaps the most important thing is to be yourself, enjoy yourself and not take yourself too seriously. If you are enjoying the class, the chances are that the students will enjoy it, too.

SUGGESTED READING

Yoga Mala by Sri K. Pattabhi Jois (North Point Press, 1999). This is the book written by Pattabhi Jois, the guru of Ashtanga yoga.

For ideas on how to modify the practice and make it safe for beginners or people with injuries: *The Practice Manual* by David Swenson (Ashtanga Yoga Productions, 2007).

For information about the poses of Ashtanga and generally how it all works and fits together: *Astanga Yoga As It Is* by Matthew Sweeney (The Yoga Temple, 2005), *Ashtanga Yoga* by Petri Räisänen (YogaWords, 2013), Ashtanga Yoga by John Scott (Gaia Books, 2000) and *Ashtanga Yoga: Practice and Philosophy* by Gregor Maehle (New World Library 2007).

For a discussion on the ethics of teaching: *Teaching Yoga: Ethics and the Teacher–Student Relationship* by Donna Farhi (Rodmell Press, 2006)

TEACHING UJJAYI BREATHING

Each school of yoga emphasises different aspects of yoga practice – for Ashtanga, a central part of the practice is the breath. The slow, deep, powerful breath is a large part of what defines Ashtanga. The aim is for the breath to be rhythmic and even, and for the movements into and out of each pose to flow along to the rhythm of the breath.

When teaching beginners it is essential continually to stress the importance of the breath. At the same time, accept that it could be months before they can coordinate movement, awareness and breath. Just keep reminding the class to breathe and repeat the breathing instructions. With more experienced students, it is surprising how often they are not using the breath properly. Use the exercises and teaching points given in this chapter, as well as suggestions and phrases you have learned from your teacher, and gently guide your students to find their ujjayi breathing.

WHY IS UJJAYI BREATHING GOOD FOR YOU?

IN YOGIC TERMS

Ujjayi breath is a form of pranayama (from the Sanskrit 'prana', meaning energy or life force, 'ayama', meaning expansion, and 'yama', meaning control). Pranayama, including ujjayi breathing, is a technique through which the quantity of energy in the body is increased and controlled.[1]

Ujjayi breathing also creates a link between the body and the mind: focusing on the sound of the breath helps to keep the practitioner in the present moment. This is important for the spiritual aspects of a yoga practice. (See Chapter 6, Teaching the Spiritual Aspects of Yoga.)

IN PHYSICAL TERMS

Breath is the most vital function of the body. If the breath is full and deep, it can positively influence the functioning of every cell. The breath is also closely connected with healthy functioning of the brain.[2]

Correct breathing allows the body to relax and open into postures or asanas. Without full, deep breathing, people can practise for years and the body will not change and open. Also, people are more likely to injure themselves when they are not breathing properly. Other specific physical areas of benefit include:

Nervous system: As described below, ujjayi breathing activates the parasympathetic nervous system, which lowers the heart rate and blood pressure, calms and relaxes the mind and encourages a feeling of connection.[3]

Circulation of blood and lymphatic fluid: Ujjayi breathing draws air into the lungs more quickly and effectively than normal breathing. This supplies oxygen to the body more efficiently and stimulates the flow of blood and lymph.[4] Stimulating blood circulation creates heat in the body. This is desirable during a yoga practice because warm muscles (like warm metal) will bend and stretch more easily and are less likely to be injured. Stimulating the lymph boosts the immune system.

Health problems: Scientific studies have indicated that ujjayi breathing can be helpful for managing depression, HIV/AIDS, the menopause, MS, insomnia and high blood pressure.[5]

BREATH AND THE NERVOUS SYSTEM

The autonomic nervous system has two components: the sympathetic, which is responsible for excitation and arousal (fight or flight); and the parasympathetic, which is responsible for relaxation (rest and digest).[6] In yoga these systems are said to correspond to the pingala and ida nadis. These nadis are lines of energy that start at the base of the spine and end in the nose. Pingala ends at the right nostril and relates to the sympathetic nervous system, and ida ends at the left nostril and relates to the parasympathetic nervous system.[7]

There is a two-way relationship between the breath and the nervous system: they affect each other. Slow, deep breathing signals to the nervous system that there is no danger and the body/mind can relax, while a relaxed body/mind will cause the breathing to become slow and deep. This means that if you deliberately deepen and slow down your breath (as in ujjayi breathing), you directly affect your body and mind through the nervous system.[8]

Muscle tension

The nervous system is part of the body's mechanism for dealing with dangerous situations. If danger is perceived, the nervous system will gear the body up for action by:

- increasing the heart rate
- stimulating adrenalin production
- decreasing normal functions such as digestion
- causing the breathing to become short and shallow
- tensing muscles ready for action

Because of the two-way relationship, shallow breathing can stimulate the fight-or-flight response. This means that the external muscles and internal muscles around the organs will become tense. So when the breath is short and shallow during an asana practice, muscles will tense and the body will not only fail to open but could actually end up tighter than it was to begin with.[9]

Stress

In an ideal situation, the sympathetic nervous system reacts in the event of danger or stress. Once the stress is resolved, the parasympathetic nervous system takes over and takes the body/mind back to a normal relaxed state.

However, the pressures and stresses of modern living often mean that we are constantly in a state of mild awareness towards danger and rarely have a chance to relax. In other words, we get stuck in the sympathetic nervous system response mode: we feel 'stressed'.

In Ashtanga yoga, the focus on the breath, and the fact that the breath is slow and deep, can take us to the parasympathetic stage: a feeling of relaxation and well-being. This is one of the mechanisms by which practising asana makes us feel better in body and mind.

CONTRAINDICATIONS

Strong ujjayi breathing may cause an adverse reaction in sufferers of low blood pressure or asthma. However, the practice can be adapted so that all students can derive benefit safely.

Low blood pressure: Ujjayi lowers blood pressure. If blood pressure is already low, then ujjayi should be practised only gently and subtly.[10] The gentle form of ujjayi could be full deep breaths with a soft 's' sound on the inhalation and an 'h' sound on the exhalation.[11]

Asthma: for people suffering from asthma, ujjayi breathing may constrict the throat too much and may contribute to breathing problems. It is best to practise a very mild ujjayi breath, and ensure the length of exhalation stays equal to the length of inhalation. Asthmatics should not attempt to flow from one posture to another in a single breath. Instead, they should add more breaths during the transitions to allow more comfortable breathing.[12]

THE FOUR STAGES

Ujjayi breath is a four-stage process:

- conscious control of the breath
- slowing and deepening the breath
- directing the breath into the upper body
- adding the ujjayi sound

CONSCIOUS CONTROL OF THE BREATH

Unconscious breath control takes place in the medulla oblongata in the primitive region of the brain. Conscious breath control takes place in the more evolved cerebral cortex. Conscious breathing therefore stimulates the functions of the more evolved areas of the brain: the neocortex and the cerebellum. The neocortex is the centre of higher order thinking, learning and memory. The cerebellum is responsible for balance, posture and coordination of movement. Conscious control of the breath can improve these functions.[13]

Conscious control of the breath forms a bridge between conscious and unconscious areas of the mind. The unconscious part of the mind is old and instinctive. It is governed by emotions. It is non-rational and unaware. It is a major force governing our reactions and behaviour. The conscious part of the brain works by a rational interpretation of our experience. If the unconscious and conscious parts of the brain do not communicate, it is easy to see how problems could develop in normal life. We will react emotionally in unthinking, non-rational ways, but at the same time react intellectually in rational thoughts. We can often end up confused and pulled in two directions. Creating a bridge between the two modes of functioning can help us to understand our reactions and decide on our actions with more clarity.[14]

SLOWING AND DEEPENING THE BREATH

Slowing and deepening the breath brings numerous physical benefits, including:

- accessing the parasympathetic nervous system, which calms the body and mind
- supplying more oxygen to the body, which enables it to function more effectively
- stimulating peristaltic action and therefore improving digestion[15]
- slowing the heart rate[16]
- lowering blood pressure[17]

By lengthening the out breath, we enable our lungs to eliminate carbon dioxide more efficiently. This can lead to a decrease in the acidity of the blood and an improvement in general health.[18]

DIRECTING THE BREATH INTO THE UPPER BODY

Upper-body, or thoracic, breathing is part of the fight-or-flight mechanism. The body/mind assumes there is danger and gears up for action.[19] This is stimulating to the nervous system, so giving energy for the yoga practice. Thoracic breathing also supplies more oxygen to muscles so they can work more effectively[20] and facilitates efficient removal of the by-products of muscles working.[21] Although they may seem contradictory, the calming, slow deep breath and stimulating thoracic breath actually balance the nervous system.

ADDING THE UJJAYI SOUND

Making the ujjayi sound gives the mind something to focus on and helps the student to become more aware of the breath, which gives them more control over their breathing.

HOW TO TEACH UJJAYI BREATHING

How you teach ujjayi will depend on how much time you have. If you are teaching a beginners' course, it is worth spending a fair amount of time covering all aspects thoroughly. If you are teaching a general drop-in class in a gym, always start by briefly setting the breath and occasionally spend longer going over breathing technique in more depth.

There are different ways to describe the breath. With beginners, it is important to pick one and stick to it. This helps to avoid confusion. I would even keep the wording consistent so it becomes an internal mental instruction. Also, keep the words you use clear and simple.

CONSCIOUS CONTROL OF THE BREATH

When teaching ujjayi breathing, the first stage is to encourage students to gain conscious awareness of the breath. Breathing usually takes place unconsciously, but we also have the ability to take conscious control. Many people new to yoga will never have been consciously aware of their breath, so it is important to start with directing awareness to the whole breathing process.

SLOWING AND DEEPENING THE BREATH

The next stage is to encourage the breath to become slower and deeper. Being aware of the breath in itself often has the effect of slowing down breathing and establishing a relaxed rhythm. There is a balance to be struck here. If the breath is too slow and deep, it can have too much of a calming effect and the energy will decrease and the heat necessary for the practice will not be generated. The breath should be slow and deep, but powerful and not too slow. For beginners it is important to talk through the process.

DIRECTING THE BREATH INTO THE UPPER BODY

For ujjayi breathing we need to breathe into the upper body (thoracic breathing). Again, beginners will often never have considered where in the body they breathe, so this will need careful explanation and demonstration.

ADDING THE UJJAYI SOUND

Once the student is aware of the breath, and has established breath that is slow and deep and directed into the chest, the last stage is to add the sound. Beginners, in particular, will need clear guidance on what kind of sound to make. Walk round the room demonstrating it so that every student has a good chance to hear it. I have found that the best way to teach the sound is to get the students to imagine they are cleaning their sunglasses (see exercise), but other ways to describe it include the wind in the trees, waves on the sea shore, a soft hissing sound, or the sound of a baby snoring (however, emphasise it is not a sniffing sound).

Some people get it straight away; others take a while. Make it clear to people having problems that it does not matter. It is a knack and they will pick it up sooner or later. They should just breathe slowly and deeply, in and out through the nose. They should neither force it nor worry about it.

Other suggestions:

Hole in the throat: Suggest students imagine they are breathing in and out through a hole in the throat (like a dolphin).

Constricting the throat: In ujjayi breathing the muscles in the throat (glottis) are lightly contracted. They are the same muscles we use when we swallow or whisper, so suggest students swallow or whisper to feel where the muscles are and then try to contract them and breathe from the throat.

Tongue to back of teeth: If you touch your tongue to the back of the front teeth where the teeth meet the gums, it engages the muscles in the throat and closes the glottis and can help to give an idea of how to make the correct ujjayi sound.

Yawning: Ujjayi breathing is a similar action to yawning, especially if you yawn with your mouth closed.

Fingers over ears: By putting the fingers over the ears, you intensify your ability to hear the breath. This will work with any of the ideas already given.

EXERCISE

STAGE ONE

CONSCIOUS CONTROL OF THE BREATH

1. Sit or lie down.
2. Become aware of the breath. Don't change it, just become aware.

TEACHING POINTS:

- Feel the breath flowing in and out of the nose.
- Do not control the breath in any way.
- Notice how the breath is cool when breathing in and warmer when breathing out.
- Observe your breath with the attitude of a detached witness.
- Feel the breath flowing in and out at the back of the mouth above the throat.
- Is the breath fast or slow?
- Is it shallow or deep?
- There is no right or wrong – you are just tuning in to what is there.

STAGE TWO

SLOWING AND DEEPENING THE BREATH

1. Lie in Savasana.
2. Focus on the breath first without changing it.
3. Begin to lengthen and deepen the breath. Start with the exhalation (because it creates a vacuum that automatically draws the inhalation into the body).

TEACHING POINTS:

- Keep the length of the inhalation equal to that of the exhalation.
- Keep the intensity of the inhalation equal to that of the exhalation.
- Breathe like this for a few minutes, then go back to normal breath.

STAGE THREE

DIRECTING THE BREATH INTO THE UPPER BODY

1. Sit or lie down and go through stages one and two, becoming aware of the breath and slowing it down.
2. Place the hands on the side of the ribcage. Breathe into the hands so that the hands move out and in again as the ribcage expands and contracts.
3. Place the hands on the chest, and breathe into them so that they move up and down as the chest rises and falls with the breath. This will help newer students check that they are breathing into the right place.
4. With a partner: sit behind your partner and place your hands on their lower ribs. Ask your partner to breathe into your hands. Then place your hands on the upper back, between the shoulder blades, and ask them to breath into your hands there.

For more advanced students, you can do this while they are practising. If you notice someone is not breathing into the upper body, place your hands on their upper back or the sides of their ribcage and give the instruction 'breathe into my hands'.

TEACHING POINTS:

- Feel how the hands move out as you breathe in.
- Keep a sense of expansion as you breathe out.

STAGE FOUR

ADDING THE UJJAYI SOUND

1. Breathing out, make a 'HA' sound as if you are breathing on your sunglasses to create a mist on the lens before wiping them.
2. Then try to make the same sound breathing in, with your mouth open. Focus on the feeling in your throat as you do this.
3. Now make the 'HA' sound breathing out and close your mouth halfway through: this is ujjayi breathing.

> 4. Finally breathe in trying to make the same sound with your mouth closed.
>
> Most students can at least get the ujjayi sound on the out-breath using this method.

GENERAL TEACHING POINTS

Once students understand the basics of breathing, you can begin to fine-tune how they use the breath in the practice. Here are some suggestions for general teaching points:

- On the inhale create space, on the exhale relax into that space.
- On the inhale lengthen, on the exhale fold.
- On the inhale lengthen, on the exhale twist.
- Keep the breath relaxed.
- Keep the face relaxed.

SUMMARY

As a teacher, make sure you breathe when you are practising and when you are teaching, especially when you are giving adjustments (see Chapter 11, Adjustments). Allow your students their learning journey with the breath, and give them support along the way.

SUGGESTED READING

For a general in-depth description of breathing in relation to yoga: *Prana, Pranayama, Prana Vidya* by Swami Niranjananada Saraswati (Yoga Publications Trust, 1994).

For clear and concise explanation of pranayama: *Asana, Pranayama, Mudra, Bandha* by Swami Satyananda Saraswati (Yoga Publications Trust, 2004).

For a look at the science behind yoga practices and clinical trials that have proved their efficacy: *Yoga As Medicine* by Timothy McCall (Bantam Books, 2007).

For an explanation of breathing specifically in relation to Ashtanga yoga: *Astanga Yoga As It Is* by Matthew Sweeney (The Yoga Temple, 2005).

For more scientific explanations: *A Textbook of Science for the Health Professions* by Barry G. Hinwood (Nelson Thornes, 1993).

TEACHING THE BANDHAS

The Sanskrit word 'bandha' means 'to hold, tighten or lock'. By 'locking' muscles on the physical level, an unlocking happens on the subtle/energetic level. By engaging physical muscles, the bandhas unlock prana (energy) and redirect its flow.

Bandhas are subtle and complicated. Matthew Sweeney interprets the meaning of the word bandha as 'binding; tying a bond, tie, chain, fetter, ligature; to catch, hold captive, arrest, imprison, fix, fasten, hold back, restrain, stop, shut, close; to redirect, clot and lock'.[22] For students and teachers alike, learning to control the bandhas is a long-term, ongoing process.

THE FOUR BANDHAS

The four bandhas are moola, uddiyana, jalandhara and maha (which is all three of the others put together). Each bandha will be applied differently depending on whether the student is practising asana or pranayama.

BENEFITS

There are three main muscle groups involved: the perineal (moola bandha), abdominal (uddiyana bandha) and cervical, or neck (jalandhara bandha). Contraction of these muscles affects the nervous, circulatory, respiratory and endocrine systems.

Nervous system: Performance of uddiyana bandha and jalandhara bandha activates the parasympathetic nervous system (the part of the nervous system that relaxes the body).[23] Moola bandha activates the sympathetic nervous system (which stimulates the body).[24] The overall effect of performing all three bandhas is to balance the nervous system,[25] which helps to regulate the body's response to internal and external stimuli.

Circulatory system: Engaging all three bandhas stimulates the circulatory system, thereby optimising the movement of oxygen, nutrients, hormones and blood around the body and the elimination of toxins and waste matter.

Respiratory system: The respiratory system comprises the airways, lungs and respiratory muscles. It introduces respiratory gases to the body and allows gaseous exchange. Engaging both the moola bandha and uddiyana bandha will directly affect breathing. These bandhas support thoracic (upper-body) breathing, which stimulates the body and prepares it for action.[26]

Endocrine system: The bandhas stimulate and balance the functioning of the endocrine system, which is a system of glands that control the body's hormonal functioning.[27] The table on page 38 summarises which bandhas affect which glands and how each gland regulates body function.

BANDHA	GLAND(S) AFFECTED	LOCATION OF GLAND	REGULATORY FUNCTION(S) OF GLAND
JALANDHARA	pineal	brain	waking and sleeping patterns
	pituitary	base of the brain	growth, blood pressure, pregnancy and childbirth, sex-organ function, thyroid-gland function, metabolism, water levels, body tempera-ture, endorphin production
	thyroid	neck	metabolism, sensitivity to other hormones
	parathyroid	on the thyroid	calcium levels (important in the functioning of the nerv-ous and muscular systems)
	thymus	behind the sternum, at the level of the heart	immune system
UDDIYANA	adrenal	above each kidney	stress response
	pancreas	just below the stomach	digestion, insulin production
MOOLA	hypothalamus	brain stem	body temperature, hunger, thirst, fatigue, sleep

Resistance: The application of the bandhas creates a kind of resistance work within the body. This engagement of muscles helps to produce heat in the body.

Stabilising the body: Muscles in the body act in pairs (for example, the biceps and the triceps). Where one muscle is engaged, the other muscle will be stabilised. By engaging the pelvic floor (moola bandha) and the lower abdominals (uddiyana bandha), we are helping to stabilise the lower back and activate the core.

Calming effect: Generally, engaging the bandhas will produce a calming effect, which lowers blood pressure and the heart rate.

CONTRAINDICATIONS

Moola bandha and uddiyana bandha should be avoided during menstruation and pregnancy, or after a heavy meal. There are no restrictions on the practice of jalandhara bandha.

MOOLA BANDHA

Moola means 'root' and moola bandha involves lifting and contracting the perineum, especially the anus. The perineum is the surface area between the thighs extending from the coccyx to the pubis; it includes the anus to the back and the external genitals to the front. Interpretations of the exact location of the bandhas vary among different yogic systems. Some systems emphasise the lift in the centre of the perineum, the Ashtanga system emphasises the lift in the anus.

For asana, we use the physical version of the bandha: lifting the anus and engaging the muscles of the perineum. For pranayama, a subtler version of moola bandha is used, and it becomes energetic.

BENEFITS

In physical terms:
- tones uro-genital and excretory functions[28]
- stimulates the nervous system via the pelvic nerves[29]
- stimulates peristalsis, which can improve digestion[30]
- helps to build core strength[31]

In yogic terms:
- sends sexual energy upwards for use as spiritual development.

HOW TO TEACH

Moola bandha is probably the hardest bandha to master and to teach. The clearest, simplest instruction is 'pelvic floor gently lifting up'. The pelvic floor is a diamond-shaped group of muscles, ligaments and fascia. It is attached to the pubis at the front, and the coccyx and sitting bones at the back. It supports the vagina, bladder and rectum and it is situated above the perineum. Moola bandha is actually more specific than a raising of the pelvic floor – it is the anus lifting up. It will be helpful to explain to beginners that if they start by engaging the pelvic floor, moola bandha will be activated and over time they will increase both awareness and control of the muscles and refine their practice of the bandha.

Women often know the location of their pelvic floor, but men often do not. You can suggest that they use the muscles normally engaged to stop a pee mid-stream. Again, this involves a larger group of muscles than moola bandha, but over time students can play with the bandha and refine it.

It is important to stress that engaging the moola bandha involves a gentle lift in the muscles. If moola bandha is practised too strongly, it can create tension in the hips, and especially in the iliopsoas (inner hip muscles). Also, explain that the buttocks should not be clenched.

EXERCISE

This exercise will help students to become more aware of the muscles around moola bandha and hopefully to gain more control.

1. Sit or lie down comfortably then relax and focus on the breath. Once breath is established, direct the focus to the whole perineal region. With each inhale and exhale, start to contract and relax this area, contracting on the inhale, and relaxing on the exhale.
2. Next, try to contract individual muscle groups: first contract the ashwini mudra (anus) and pulse the contraction with the breath. Then, isolate and contract the vajroli mudra (muscles that stop your pee), pulsing the contraction with the breath.
3. Finally, see if you can isolate the part in the centre between the anus and genitals.

TEACHING POINTS:

- Feel your pelvic floor gently lifting up.
- Feel a lift in the anus.

UDDIYANA BANDHA

From the Sanskrit for 'flying up', uddiyana bandha is the engagement of the lower abdominal muscles – more specifically, the part of the abdominal wall between the two hip bones (anterior superior iliac spines). During pranayama, this bandha is engaged strongly with external breath retention (holding the breath after exhalation). While practising asana, we use a subtler version.

BENEFITS

In physical terms:

- stimulates digestion[32]
- stimulates blood circulation[33]
- strengthens abdominal muscles[34]
- helps to access core strength[35]
- balances adrenals[36]

In yogic terms:

- keeps energy rising upwards

HOW TO TEACH

To teach the full bandha used for pranayama:

- Stand with your feet apart, bend the knees and bend forward at the waist.
- Rest your hands on your thighs just above the knee with the arms straight.
- Breathe all the air out of your lungs in a 'whoosh' through your mouth.
- Tuck your chin down to your chest, curve the spine forwards and make a false inhalation, expanding the chest as though you are breathing in but keeping the glottis closed so you do not take in any air. The abdominal muscles should draw right up but stay soft.

To teach the version for asana:

This is the subtler version of the bandha. The clearest instruction is 'lower abdominal muscles gently lifting in and up'.

It is also helpful to instruct your class to try different asana both with and without uddiyana bandha. This way students can experience the difference. Try some twists and use uddiyana bandha on the exhalation to go deeper or more comfortably into the twist.

EXERCISE

This seated variation is a gentle introduction to uddiyana bandha. It is particularly suitable for beginners, who may well need some time to practise this bandha.

---

1. Sit comfortably, gently breathing into the stomach.
2. Place your hands on the lower abdominals between the hip bones. Feel how your hands move with your breath.
3. Create a gentle lift in the lower abdominals so your hands move in and up about 2.5cm. This is uddiyana bandha.
4. Hold that lift and carry on breathing normally. Notice what happens to the movement in your abdomen and chest. The abdomen should move less and the chest more.

TEACHING POINTS:

- Lower abdominals gently lift in and up.
- As the abdominals move in and up, the front of the ribcage should not move up too. It should stay fairly still.

JALANDHARA BANDHA

Jalandhara means 'net in the stream'. Jalandhara bandha is the movement of drawing the chin down towards the chest. The full performance of this bandha involves holding the breath (either by holding the breath in or out). Because we never hold the breath in asana practice, we do not perform the full version of jalandhara bandha in asana classes. A subtler version of jalandhara bandha is used to keep the back of the neck long.

BENEFITS

In physical terms:
- improves the function of the veins and nerves that feed the brain
- rebalances the neck muscles and bones (incorrectly positioning the head can create tension in the muscles on the front of the neck and contract the muscles at the back of the neck)
- stimulates the thyroid and helps balance its functioning, thereby regulating the metabolism[37]

In yogic terms:
- focuses the mind
- helps energy to flow freely

HOW TO TEACH

To teach the version for pranayama:

- Sit comfortably, breathe deeply.
- Inhale or exhale slowly and deeply, and hold the breath.
- Keeping the back of the neck long, gently bring the chin down towards the chest. Make sure you do not sink the chest down, too.
- Hold for as long as comfortable.
- Release the head, then breathe.

To teach the version for asana:

- The clearest instructions are 'draw the chin down towards the chest' or 'keep the back of the neck long'.
- To demonstrate to students the importance of the back of the neck being long, have the students do several asana such as Parsvottanasana (see page 203) and Trikonasana (see pages 196–7) and explore the positioning of the head. It should feel much nicer to have the head positioned correctly.

MAHA BANDHA AND NAULI

MAHA BANDHA

Maha ('great') bandha is the action of performing all three individual bandhas at once.

To access maha bandha:

- Sit comfortably, close the eyes and breathe slowly.
- Breathe all the air out of the lungs and hold the breath.
- Apply jalandhara, uddiyana and moola bandhas in that order. Hold the bandhas for as long as it is comfortable, then release moola, uddiyana and jalandhara bandhas in that order.
- Slowly inhale.

NAULI

Although not actually a bandha, nauli is often performed in conjunction with uddiyana bandha before practising Ashtanga yoga. It involves a rolling of the abdominal muscles, which helps to improve digestive function. As is the case for moola bandha and uddiyana bandha, nauli should be avoided by women when they are menstruating or pregnant (or trying to become pregnant) and by anyone who has recently eaten a heavy meal.

To perform nauli:

- Stand with the feet hip-width apart, fold forwards at the waist, rest your hands on the thighs just above the knees and perform full uddiyana bandha.
- Next, move one of your hands away from the thighs so you are now resting your weight on just one hand. The stomach muscles on that side of the abdomen should engage and stick out to the side.
- Play with the possibility of shifting from one hand resting on the thigh to the other, so engaging the muscles alternately on each side of the abdomen.
- Once you can do this comfortably, explore pushing the centre of the abdominals downwards in a ridge as you swap from one side to the other, so the abdominal muscles appear to roll.
- Draw the abdominal muscles back up as you swap back.

GENERAL TEACHING POINTS

Explain to your students that holding energetic locks or bandhas while practising physical postures will help to keep their energy rising. The bandhas also help to protect the spine and lower-back muscles, which can be fragile.

- Moola bandha: pelvic floor (or anus) gently lifting up.
- Uddiyana bandha: lower abdominals gently lifting in and up.
- Jalandhara bandha: back of the neck long.

Stress that the bandhas should be held lightly: if they are engaged too strongly, they can create restrictions within the body and in the breath, which is counterproductive.

BANDHAS IN ASHTANGA

The bandhas are not constantly engaged for the whole duration of our practice. The action is more subtle than that. The bandhas will come and go in intensity depending on the asana you are practising. Bandhas pass back and forth, never fully locking and never fully letting go. The bandhas flow with the breath: moola bandha works more strongly on the exhalation and uddiyana bandha on the inhalation. Some people believe the opposite is true: try them both ways and see what you think.

As an exercise, do a whole practice and focus only on the bandhas: moola bandha on the exhalation and uddiyana bandha on the inhalation. Teach a whole class just focused on the bandhas and breath in the same way.

SUMMARY

Your understanding of bandhas in your teaching and practice will change and evolve over the years. Stress to beginners that they are not expected to get everything perfect straightaway. Explain to more experienced students that bandhas are something to work on, explore and experiment with.

SUGGESTED READING

For clear explanations and clear instructions on how to do bandhas: *Asana, Pranayama, Mudra, Bandha* by Swami Satyananda Saraswati (Yoga Publications Trust, 2004).

For a scientific and fairly academic take on bandhas: *Anatomy of Hatha Yoga* by David Coulter (Body and Breath, 2001).

For more on anatomy: *Yoga Anatomy* by Leslie Kaminoff (The Breathe Trust, 2007). This book also has very clear anatomical information for many of the poses in the Primary Series.

TEACHING THE DRISTI

Each posture has a dristi or gaze point. The eyes look towards this point – you do not necessarily have to actually see or focus on the point. The dristi have numerous yogic and physical benefits. For example, they enable us to maintain focus and concentration, help us to balance and improve eye health.

When teaching a led class, always mention the dristi as you talk students into each posture and keep reminding them to hold the dristi steady. As with all actions in yoga, the gaze should be light and never forced. It is the three-fold attention on breath, bandhas and dristi that transforms a physical practice into something deeper.

THE NINE DRISTI

There are nine dristi in total:

Nasagrai dristi – look to the nose
Urdhva dristi – look straight up
Ajna dristi – look to the third eye (at the top of the nose,
    in between the eyebrows)
Hastagrai dristi – look to the hand
Angustha Madyai dristi – look to the thumb
Parsva dristi – look to the right
Parsva dristi – look to the left
Nabi dristi – look to the navel
Padayaragrai dristi – look to the foot[38]

Generally, when the action moves upwards, the gaze also is directed upwards. Similarly, when the body folds down, the gaze is directed downwards. One exception to this principle is backbends, during which the dristi is normally directed towards the nose (nasagrai dristi). The table on pages 49–51 itemises which dristi should be used with each pose.

BENEFITS

Maintains focus: The dristi keeps the attention internal and reduces distractions. When we are looking around, it is obviously much harder to maintain focus and very easy to get distracted.

Stimulates nervous system: When the eyes are looking around, the nervous system receives signals that there might be danger. The sympathetic nervous system is consequently stimulated and both the body and the mind prepare for action. If the eyes remain still, the parasympathetic system is stimulated, and both the body and mind relax.[39]

Tells you which way to stretch: In each posture there are several different directions in which we can stretch. Generally, we should stretch towards the direction of our gaze. Therefore, the dristi normally offers guidance on which way to go.

Helps balance: There are muscles in the body that respond to the movement of the eyes. The body unconsciously expects to follow the eyes, so these muscles get ready to move when the eyes move. If you place your thumbs under the occipital ridge at the back of the neck, then move the eyes from side to side, you will feel the engagement of the muscles in the neck as they get ready to move. So the dristi can help the body stretch in a pose and it can also help to maintain balance in balancing poses.

Improves eye health: The eyes are affected by two sets of muscles. First, the internal muscles, which control the position and shape of the lens within the eye – these are really the most important muscles in terms of how well we see. Second, the external muscles, which control the movement of the whole eye – these are the muscles affected by the dristi. These muscles can have a negative effect on vision and the health of the eyes if they are stiff and weak. The dristi works these muscles and ensures they are as flexible and strong as possible.[40]

EYE EXERCISES

To feel the full effect of the dristi, it is good to practise them in isolation.

1. Sit comfortably. First do some palming: rub the hands together until they are hot, then cup the hands so the palms are over but not touching the eyes. Remove the hands from the eyes.
2. For five seconds each: look up, down, right, left, up-right, down-right, up-left, down-left. Rotate several times one way then the other.
3. Hold a thumb arms' length away and focus on the tip of the nose for two seconds. Focus on the thumb for two seconds, then shift your focus to another point further away for two seconds. Repeat this sequence several times.
4. Repeat the palming.

TABLE OF DRISTI AND POSES

The following table shows the dristi for the major salutations and standing, sitting and finishing poses. Note that there is not necessarily one absolutely correct dristi. It seems that different dristi have been taught to different people at different times. The important thing is that you have a dristi; it doesn't necessarily matter exactly where it is. If you find the 'correct' dristi a strain, then choose another one. I have given alternatives for poses where the dristi can be challenging or where different ways are commonly taught. Looking to the nose and the third eye can be difficult at first, so advise students to try doing it for a short while and build it up slowly. Looking to the nose can be replaced with looking down, and looking up can replace the third eye.

POSE	DRISTI
SUN SALUTATIONS	
Surya Namaskara A	
inhale – reach up	third eye or hand
exhale – fold down	nose
inhale – lift the chest	third eye
exhale – Chatturanga	nose
inhale – up dog	nose or third eye
exhale – down dog	navel, nose or the back edge of your mat
Surya namaskara B	
inhale – Virabhadrasana 1	third eye or hand
STANDING POSES	
Padangushtasana	nose
Utthita and Parivrtta Trikonasana	hand
Utthita and Parivrtta Parsvakonasana	hand
Prasarita Padottanasana	nose
Parsvottanasana	big toe or nose
Utthita Hasta Padangushtasana	
first part	foot, off the end of the nose, or floor
second part	side or floor
third part	nose or floor
Ardha Baddha Padmottanasana	nose or floor
Utkatasana	hand
Virabhadrasana I and II	hand

SITTING POSES	
Dandasana	nose or toes
Paschimattanasana	nose
Purvattanasana	nose
Ardha Baddha Padma Paschimattanasana	foot
Tiriangamukhaikapada Paschimattanasana	foot
Janu Sirsasana A, B and C	foot
Marichyasana A	foot
Marichyasana B	nose
Marichyasana C	side
Marichyasana D	side
Navasana	nose or toes
Bhujapidasana	nose
Kurmasana	third eye
Supta Kurmasana	nose
Garbha Pindasana	nose
Baddha Konasana	nose
Upavishta Konasana	
first part	nose
second part	upwards
Supta Konasana	navel
Supta Padangushtasana	
first part	foot
second part	side
Ubhaya Padangushtasana	upwards
Urdvha Mukha Paschimattanasana	nose or feet
Setu Bandhasana	nose
FINISHING POSES	
Urdhva Dhanurasana	nose
Paschimattanasana	foot
Salamba Sarvangasana	navel
Matsyasana	nose

Uttana Padasana	nose
Sirsasana	nose
Balasana	eyes closed
Baddha Padmasana	nose
Yoga Mudra	third eye
Padmasana	nose
Uth Pluthi	nose

SUMMARY

The dristi works in conjunction with the breath and bandhas to deepen yoga practice (this is the idea of Tristana, the three-fold attention on breath, bandha and dristi). It helps to focus the mind, as well as improving balance and strengthening eye muscles. Each pose has one or more suggested dristi, which usually correspond to the direction of the movement in the pose.

SUGGESTED READING

For clear explanations and instructions on how to do dristi: *Asana, Pranayama, Mudra, Bandha* by Swami Satyananda Saraswati (Yoga Publications Trust, 2004).

For explanations of dristi in relation to Ashtanga yoga: *Astanga Yoga As It Is* by Matthew Sweeney (The Yoga Temple, 2005).

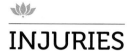

INJURIES

When we take on any kind of physical activity, we run the risk that injuries may occur. As a teacher, it is your responsibility to create an environment that is based not on striving towards goals but on paying attention to the body. You should also explain the different sensations in the body: the difference between safe stretching and damaging pain.

However, even when every precaution has been taken, some of your students may still hurt themselves – or you may hurt yourself – and it is important that you know how to deal with different kinds of injury.

CAUSES OF INJURY

OLD INJURIES

Scar tissue is less flexible than normal healthy muscle fibres. If a muscle with scar tissue is stretched, the healthy fibres in the muscle will start to stretch, but the scar tissue in the muscle will not, and this can cause tearing. When this happens, it is an opportunity to re-heal the injury in a healthier way (see page 57, Working With An Existing Injury).

POINTS OF WEAKNESS

Weak points are more susceptible to injury. It is good practice as a teacher to be aware of your students' specific weak points, and to adapt the practice to safeguard against exacerbating those weak points. For instance, if a student has a weak back, you could suggest they use their bandhas strongly when going into and out of forward bends and teach the student strengthening exercises for the back.

BAD HABITS

It is important that students take responsibility for their practice. Injuries do not just happen; we normally do something to cause them to happen. Examples of bad habits displayed by certain students include pushing too hard or maintaining a bad posture.

Pushing too hard

New students will often try to push or pull themselves further into a posture. However, pushing or pulling into a posture is more likely to cause the body to tense, and practising yoga with tense muscles is likely to result in injury. For example, pulling into a forward bend using the arms will create shoulder tension, which is counterproductive. It is better to engage the uddiyana bandha and use the exhalation to go deeper into the fold. Therefore, the role of the teacher is to stress the importance of relaxing, softening and breathing, rather than pushing and pulling.

Bad posture

Common examples of bad posture are:

breath or holding the breath signals to the nervous system to tense up, so if a student breathes in this way the muscles will tense and injury is much more likely. There is a balance to be struck here, though, because if the breath becomes too slow then the heat and energy needed for an Ashtanga practice won't be generated. (See Chapter 2, Teaching Ujjayi Breathing.)

Awareness: Always tell students to err on the side of caution when practising with pain, and focus on developing the student's awareness of their 'edge'. The edge is the place where the student feels a gentle stretch and just before they start to feel pain. Once they are at the edge, the key is to relax and breathe, to explore and play – not to push and strain. If pain is persistent, there are several options. Firstly, the asana can be modified so the pain is avoided – for example, by sitting on a block. If modification is not possible, the student may have to stop practising this asana for a while.

ADJUSTMENTS

Although adjustments are a powerful tool for improving your students' practice, they can also be a potential cause of injury if not performed correctly. The most important thing is clear communication between teacher and student.

Trust and communication: Ask permission before making an adjustment on a student and remind your students that they are allowed to refuse. Always respect when a student says 'no'. Make sure your students understand that they have the right – and responsibility – to tell you straightaway if an adjustment is too strong, rather than putting up with it. If you are not sure, ask if the adjustment is too much.

Resistance: Sometimes when giving an adjustment, you cannot feel resistance but the student feels pain. In this scenario, you should stop the adjustment. In other cases, you can feel resistance but it feels good for the student for you to push gently through it. If you intend to push through resistance, it is extremely important that you check with the student if it feels all right.

Breath: Watch the student's body carefully. If you cannot see evidence of conscious deep breathing, do not make an adjustment. If, halfway through the adjustment, the student's breath becomes shallow or the muscles start to shake, back off.

If you do injure someone: Take responsibility. Apologise and explain what happened from your point of view. Make sure you have insurance (see Chapter 1, Teaching Yoga).

WORKING WITH AN EXISTING INJURY

As well as preventing new injuries, you will also need to deal with students' existing injuries and know how to avoid making them worse. If someone comes to your class with an injury and you are unsure whether it is safe for the student to practise, ask them to speak to their GP first. Always ask when they injured themselves. If the injury is very recent (within the last 48 hours), if there is redness or swelling, or if it is very painful, the student should not practise. Inexperienced students who haven't learned to tell the difference between damaging pain and safely stretching a muscle should in any case probably rest until their injury has healed.

If the injury is old, most students can work around it. Always tell them not to do anything that hurts, especially if they experience sharp pain. As the class proceeds, show the injured student how to modify postures to protect the injured area. Ask them at the end how the injury feels. If it feels worse then you need to decide if it is best for them not to do yoga again until the injury heals or if they need to modify more and be more careful next time. Be firm: if you feel that a student's injury cannot be worked around, tell the student to stop practising completely until it has healed.

Be especially careful with knee injuries. If the meniscus is injured, then a student should not do anything that causes pain. Knees can take a long time to heal – years even – but if they are treated with care, they can heal over time.

DEALING WITH A NEW INJURY

If someone sustains an injury in your class, attend to them immediately and make sure they are comfortable and warm enough. If necessary, stop the class to look after them. Put ice on the injury (if appropriate) and follow the other first-aid steps given below. Make sure there is a first-aid kit in the place where you teach, and ensure that you know how to use it.

If you are teaching in a gym or a yoga centre, it is the owner's responsibility to make sure there is a qualified first-aider on hand and a fully stocked first-aid kit, but it is worth checking that they have dealt with this. If you have hired a hall, then you need to make sure you have assessed any risks to your own or your students' health and safety and made your environment safe. For further information, consult the Health and Safety Executive (HSE) website and also the International Yoga Teachers' Association Occupational Health and Safety

Guidelines. You are also required to provide your own 'adequate and appropriate' first-aid equipment. This means a first-aid box and someone who knows how to use it. The HSE website gives basic advice on administering first aid in case of an emergency. This is not a substitute to doing a first-aid course, but it may help to jog your memory if something does go wrong.

FIRST AID FOR MUSCLE INJURIES

The acronym RICE stands for Rest, Immobilise, Cold (or Compression), Elevate. This is a handy way to remember the first-aid treatment for a muscle tear or strain.

Rest

The student should rest an acute injury for at least 48 hours, especially if there is swelling or redness. They should not have any massage or bodywork, as massage on a freshly torn muscle can make the tearing worse. If the muscle has gone into spasm, then gentle massage can help.

Immobilise

If you are not sure what kind of injury it is, then err on the side of caution and advise the student to leave their body to do the initial healing and keep the injured area as still as possible.

Cold

Ice works in two ways. First, icing constricts the blood vessels, which reduces internal bleeding. Second, when the blood vessels contract then expand again, they flush fresh blood and lymphatic fluid through the injured area, which speeds up the healing process.

How to apply an ice pack:
- Wrap the ice in a thin cloth and apply to the affected area. Do not apply ice directly to the skin.
- Leave ice on the body for no longer than five minutes. After about five minutes, the nervous system starts reacting as if the body is being frozen and sends signals to heat up the area, which counteracts the benefits of the ice.
- Leave the skin until it returns to its normal temperature (normally

around 33°C, but this can vary depending on external conditions).
- Reapply ice onto the skin.
- Advise the student to keep regularly icing the injury for at least a few days. They should apply ice especially after taking exercise that uses the injured area.

Ice will not help if the muscle has gone into spasm rather than sustained a tear. Spasm means that the muscle has contracted and cannot relax. If a muscle is in spasm, heat treatment is more likely to help to relax it. For a heat treatment, follow the instructions above but substitute the ice pack for a heat pack or hot water bottle.

Elevation

While there is swelling, the injured person should lie down as often as possible, and raise the injury above the heart. This will help the swelling go down.

FIRST AID FOR SHOCK

Although it is unlikely that anything you do in your classes will cause a student to go into shock, it is such a serious condition that it is important you know what to do if it does arise. Medical shock is when the tissues in the body don't receive enough oxygen and nutrients to allow the cells to function. Treatment given in the early stages of shock is particularly significant; if untreated, it leads to whole-body failure and death. Shock can be caused by (among other things) heart attack, anaemia, excessive bleeding, low blood sugar, allergic reaction or extreme dehydration. The symptoms are cool clammy skin, weak and rapid pulse, nausea, lifeless eyes, and a weak and confused mental state. If you suspect shock, first call an ambulance. Then have the person lie down on their back with feet about 30cm higher than the head. If raising the legs is likely to cause pain or further injury, keep them flat. Keep the person still, warm and comfortable, soothe and reassure them, and do not give them anything by mouth.

TYPES OF JOINT INJURY

So that you treat them appropriately, it can be helpful to understand the symptoms of different kinds of joint injury. However, if you are in any doubt, seek the advice of a qualified physiotherapist or GP.

Injuries to ligaments: You will experience sharp pain and swelling at the time of the injury. Follow the instructions for a new injury. Then, do not use the joint if it hurts. The key is to work on strengthening rather than stretching the joint once the initial swelling/heat has gone down.

Injuries to tendons: These tend to give sharp pain at the time of injury but without the swelling associated with ligament injuries. Again, follow the instructions for a new injury, and then work on gently stretching the joint in the pain-free range.

Injuries to muscles: If you become aware of pain the next day and there was no specific incident that may have caused the injury, then the pain is probably the result of muscle strain.

REHABILITATION

Once the injury has had the initial 48 hours of rest, as long as any swelling or redness has gone down, it is important to start moving it again. Initially, it should be worked very gently and in the pain-free-range. If an injury is rested too long, the area may heal with internal scar tissue. This will mean that flexibility and strength can be permanently lost and the area will be prone to being re-injured.

Often the muscles around an injured area will tense up. This is the body immobilising the area to protect itself. These muscles often need to be gently massaged to release after the injury.

It takes a great deal of patience and awareness to work safely with an injury, but it can be done and the injured person will learn a lot about their body, their yoga practice and perhaps their attitude to both.

Complementary remedies

Arnica can be taken internally as a homeopathic remedy (arnica 200 once an hour for a day then once a day after that for as long as necessary). It can also be applied to the injury (so long as the skin is not broken) as a cream, oil or tincture. The essential oils of lavender and chamomile can help with bruising (dilute in a carrier oil – refer to instructions on the bottle).

SUMMARY

Dealing with injuries as a yoga teacher is a problematic area. However, if you use these guidelines and your common sense and always proceed with caution, it can be very satisfying to help a student heal an injury or learn to accommodate it within their practice.

TEACHING THE SPIRITUAL ASPECTS OF YOGA

A book on teaching yoga would be incomplete without mentioning how to teach yoga's spiritual aspects. This is a difficult topic for many reasons. Firstly, yogic philosophy is a vast – and complex – field. It spans thousands of years and takes in a huge range of different perspectives and viewpoints. Secondly, in order to teach something, you really need to understand it yourself and have a fairly clear idea of what you think and feel about the issues. It can often take years of study and thought to begin to know what you believe and what it means to live by your beliefs. Thirdly, spirituality can be a very sensitive subject for students. Some people may feel that yoga's spiritual aspects interfere with their own spiritual practice, or that they challenge or imply disrespect to their beliefs. However, other people may be highly resistant to any 'spirituality' talk, especially any mention of God. It is obviously important not to preach. Equally, though, you would be leaving out a huge component of yoga if you were never to mention spirituality at all.

In this chapter, I offer my ideas about the spiritual aspects of yoga and how to incorporate them into an Ashtanga yoga class. My hope as a teacher is to spark students' interest, and to inspire them to discover yoga philosophy for themselves.

YOGA PRACTICE AS NEUTRAL

A yoga practice, especially an asana practice, can be entirely neutral from the standpoint of belief. If you practise yoga, you do not have to subscribe to any particular faith or belief. So a yoga practitioner can see the practice as purely physical, something that makes them healthier physically and happier emotionally. Or a student can take the feeling of clarity and peace that yoga provides and use it to deepen an existing religious or spiritual practice, such as Christianity or Islam. Or a yoga practice can be a complete spiritual path in itself, independent of any external religious framework. (I am making a distinction here between 'religions', with their specific trappings and belief systems, and more universal principles about what lies beyond the purely material.)

Personally, I came to yoga for purely physical reasons. However, over the years I found more and more that interested me under the broad umbrella of yoga philosophy. The vast, diverse and sometimes apparently contradictory teachings of yoga philosophy have contributed to my self-understanding, and helped me live my life in a happier way. The spiritual process tends to start to happen to people anyway when they practise asana, but learning the philosophy can give a student a clearer framework for what is happening and so help the process along. What is meant by 'philosophy' here may be different from the usual meaning of the word in the West, because yoga philosophy is oriented to a practical goal and to spiritual ends.

DEFINING SPIRITUALITY

Firstly, it is important to define 'spiritual'. Most dictionary definitions refer to a belief in something 'other than the purely material or mechanical'. But as a teacher you really have to think about what you mean. If you talk about a 'spiritual path' or 'spiritual practice' or 'developing spiritually', what do you mean?

I see spirituality as incorporating some kind of inner transformation, whereby a student gains a higher sense of clarity and peace, bringing in turn a greater feeling of freedom and connection.

In this chapter I have divided yogic spirituality into five areas:

Focus: In order for spiritual development to happen, the mind needs to become still. If the mind is forever chattering, reviewing the past, anticipating the future, criticising our self and others, then spiritual transformation is not going to take place. This stillness is gained primarily through focus, so first we will examine how Ashtanga yoga helps us to gain focus and how you can incorporate it into an Ashtanga class.

Clarity: The mind also needs to become freer from unthinking patterns and neuroses. These stop us from seeing things as they really are and reacting from a place of clarity and truth. So secondly we will consider Ashtanga yoga as therapy, and see how Ashtanga can help us to identify these patterns and start to transcend them.

Happiness: As well as helping us to develop spiritually, yoga practice can also make us happier, and 'happiness' is a concept that is perhaps easier than 'spirituality' for many students to take on board initially. So next we will explore the idea of happiness and how it relates to yoga.

Yogic concepts: Next we will look at how key ethical principles contained within the Yoga Sutras – the foundation of classical yoga – relate to Ashtanga and how you can start to incorporate them in your classes.

Yoga as energy: Finally, we will think about the hatha yoga tradition, in which the postures are viewed as a spiritual practice in themselves and are considered to generate subtle energy through the interaction of the physical body and the energetic body.

This is not an exhaustive list. There are many other angles you can take, but hopefully this will give you some ideas to start with and help you to develop your own.

HOW TO TEACH SPIRITUALITY

Sometimes as a teacher you will be addressing the whole class in general terms, but you should also be prepared to talk about spirituality more personally with individual students.

To the whole class: When you are talking to the whole class, introduce your theme near the beginning of the session. Remind the students several times during the class, and then sum up at the end. It is also a good idea to suggest ways the students can bring these ideas into their daily life. Yoga is not just something we do in a yoga class; it is something that can continue throughout our entire lives. The lessons we learn about ourselves in our yoga practice normally apply to ourselves in the rest of our lives.

To individual students: When you are talking to individual students, listen carefully to what they say and what questions they ask, and try to work out what information will be helpful to them. It is fairly common for students to start feeling the spiritual aspects of yoga, the clarity and peace and sense of well-being, and for them to ask their teacher about it. Generally, it is helpful to explain to them that this is an important aspect of yoga. If they want to do some reading, recommend a translation of the Yoga Sutras and suggest they start by reading about the yamas and niyamas. Some books focus specifically on these areas (see Suggested Reading, pages 80–1).

FOCUS: STILLING THE MIND

Focus is something concrete. It's something you can do, especially in a yoga class. Spirituality cannot be approached directly; you have to come at it with the tool of focused awareness. It is normally obvious when someone has decided to become 'more spiritual' – there is something forced and false about them. It is also obvious when someone has had a spiritual practice for a long time: their eyes shine and they seem relaxed and happy within themselves.

The focus stemming from a yoga practice leads to a quieting of the mind. This means that the usual chatter and commentary that many of us have running through our minds becomes less intrusive. Once this chatter starts to diminish, then we can start to think and see more clearly. Essentially, focus is about getting the chattering or 'discursive' mind out of the way.

FOCUS AND ASHTANGA

One criticism often levelled at Ashtanga yoga is that it is not spiritual, it is 'just gymnastics'. I have also heard yoga teachers state that if you do not believe in God then you are just doing gymnastics.

Firstly, anything can be spiritual – including gymnastics. If someone is doing something with absolute focus, wholly absorbed and fully in the present, then this can lead to spiritual development. It can be virtually anything: often it is something a person is good at, something they enjoy. It may be something creative or physical, like playing music, dancing, painting or playing football. God does not have to be involved at all. Many strands of yogic philosophy, including samkhya, which is the philosophical base for the Yoga Sutras, do not include any idea of God (although the Yoga Sutras themselves do).

Secondly, Ashtanga yoga is particularly well suited to creating this feeling of focus. The fact that it is practised in a set sequence of poses means that the mind can switch off from everyday thoughts. We can become absorbed and flowing without the need to think about what we are doing.

You could easily do a practice that looks more spiritual, like sitting and chanting 'Om' in a white robe, but if you are thinking about what's for tea it's not spiritual at all.

TEACHING FOCUS

Talking about focus is an accessible way of bringing up the spiritual aspects of yoga during your classes. Explain to your students that one of the things yoga is aiming to achieve is stilling the mind and that we do this primarily through focus. There are several ways to talk about focus that can enable you to briefly mention an aspect of yoga philosophy, or a more advanced aspect of asana practice. These will hopefully not put off students who are resistant to the idea of spirituality and might catch the interest of students who are more open to the ideas.

Yoga Sutras

- Start the class by explaining that yoga is not just about the body, it is about the mind, too.
- The Ashtanga yoga chant acknowledges Patañjali, who was one of the first people to write about yoga in a systematic way.
- Mention that some form of yoga has been practised for around 4,000 years and that Patañjali wrote the Yoga Sutras around 2,000 years ago. (Estimated periods of time vary widely among commentators. These are average estimates.)
- Near the beginning of Patañjali's text we read *yogaschitta vrtti nirodhah*, which can be translated as 'yoga is stilling the fluctuations of the mind'. In addition to increasing strength and flexibility in our bodies through yoga, we are also stilling our minds so we can feel clearer and be more peaceful.
- We still our minds through focus. By keeping our focus on the body and the breath, our mind is kept in the present moment.
- Throughout the class come back to the idea of focus and what is happening in the mind.

Union

- Start the class by talking about the meaning of the word 'yoga', which is often translated as 'union'.
- This union works on many levels.
- The first level is union of the body and the mind.
- An easy way to access this is to focus the mind on the breath.
- The breath is a bridge between the body and the mind.
- By focusing on the breath we bring peace and clarity to the mind.

Dristi

- Start the class by talking about dristi, or gaze points (see Chapter 4, Teaching the Dristi).
- One of the reasons why we use dristi is to keep the mind focused.
- The reason we want to keep the mind focused is to gain a sense of peace and clarity, which is ultimately what yoga is all about.
- And again throughout the class come back to the dristi and the sense of focus.

Breath

- Start the class by talking about the breath.
- We do a special kind of breathing for many reasons, one of which is to help us keep our focus.
- Keep coming back to the idea of focus on the sound of the breath, which leads to peace and clarity.

Teaching points

- Ask the question 'where is your focus?'
- Give the instruction 'gently bring the focus back to the body and the breath'.
- Every now and then, during the standing postures, instruct the class to stop in Tadasana with the eyes closed. Ask the students to focus on the feeling of:
  o   the breath, and how it moves the body

o   the air on their skin

o   the mat under their feet

o   their heart beating

CLARITY: YOGA AS THERAPY

Like focus, clearing the mind of unhelpful, unconscious patterns is something you can work on. A yoga practice can help you to clear your mind and you need to do this before a deep spiritual transformation can happen. Explain to your students that a yoga practice can help them to see things more clearly and react more openly from a space of truth and honesty rather than simply reacting without thinking and acting out old patterns of behaviour.

CLARITY AND ASHTANGA

To develop spiritually, to be truly clear and at peace, it is not enough to cultivate focus and concentration if underneath the focus we are a mass of neuroses. A yoga practice can help us sort out the issues that prevent us from seeing the world as it is and reacting intelligently and appropriately. Every day when we step onto our mats, we enter a space where how we act and what we think and feel about others and ourselves is magnified and mirrored back to us. The practice itself is neutral, but it will show very clearly what our patterns are. For example, if you tend to push yourself too hard, always give up, become competitive, blame other people or get jealous, then a yoga practice will show up these traits. You then have the option to recognise the pattern, admit it and deal with it.

One issue I dealt with was the habit of comparing myself to other people and deciding whether I was 'better' or 'worse' than them. After practising for a while, I realised that there would always be people more able than I at asana and people less able. Where then does all that comparing leave me? Nowhere! Let it go! Gain that mental space for some peace and quiet. It's not that I no longer feel the emotion, but I can observe it from a place of discernment and not be controlled by it. This is close to the yogic ideal of *upeksha*, or equanimity. It's not that you are no longer passionate about life, or don't feel things strongly any more, but you have the choice about how to act on these emotions and issues.

TEACHING CLARITY

Talk about these issues during the sitting poses. Forward bends are naturally inward-looking poses and often a time in the practice when a beginner student's attention can start to wander.

Patterns of behaviour

One fairly simple tool you can use as a yoga teacher is to talk about unconscious patterns of behaviour and how we can use our yoga practice to learn about ourselves and perhaps find more balance and happiness. The following points may help you to structure your discussion:

- There are two clear patterns in a yoga practice. When things get tough, some people respond by pushing themselves extremely hard, while others give up. Try pointing out those two patterns and suggest that the students observe themselves to see if they fall into one of the two patterns. Point out that if that is how they react during their yoga practice, then it is probably how they react in the rest of their lives.
- Suggest to your students that once they have noticed their pattern, that they try to find the middle ground where they respond to challenges in a way that is healthy and productive. This means trying, but not too hard. In the yoga posture they find their edge and then relax and allow change to happen.

This is really about learning to listen to our inner voice, our intuition. What is right for us? If we can learn to listen during our yoga practice, then maybe we can learn to listen in the rest of our lives.

Negative thought patterns

Explain to your students that one of the things we are aiming to achieve through yoga is clarity of the mind. Most of us have thoughts that come into the mind and disturb the stillness. It can be useful to notice what those thoughts are, because by noticing them we can start to see our patterns and start to let them go. Do they fall into a category? Common patterns are:

- worrying about things that might happen in the future
- going over the past

- mentally writing a list of things to do
- criticising ourselves and others

You could point out that worrying about things that might happen is not really helpful. If there is something you can do to help sort out a problem in your life, then do it. If there's nothing you can do about it, then worrying is certainly not going to help. What's more, you can't know what's going to happen in the future. The thing you're worrying about might never happen, so worrying about it is a complete waste of time.

Similarly, going over the past is a waste of time, because what is done is done. If you have done something you feel unhappy about, then take action to resolve the mistake or regret. If there is nothing you can do, then worrying about it is not going to help: it will just make you feel bad.

Writing a list of things to do can be constructive, but a yoga class is not the best time to do it: we're trying to quieten the mind, rather than analyse our life.

Criticising ourselves and others will only take us into spirals of negative feeling.

We do have control over our thoughts. If you notice a thought pattern that makes you unhappy, whenever it comes, as soon as you notice it, let it go. Giving thoughts time and attention feeds them and makes them stronger, and more likely to return. If you consciously let them go, they will fade away. It may take a while, but this technique can work.

Sometimes, when confronted by a painful thought, ask yourself: is it really true? How does the thought make you feel? Is the complete opposite of that thought also true? In some cases a deeper understanding of the particular issue is needed. This is often the case with deep-seated emotional scars. In these cases, you might address these issues outside of class. Ask yourself if your thoughts and mental patterns help you, or increase your happiness? If the answer is 'no', then take these steps to change them:

- As before, the first step is awareness. What is your predominant thought pattern?
- Then comes acceptance. It is important that we do not judge ourselves for having these thought patterns: after all, everyone has them.
- The next step is investigation. Where does the pattern come

from? Are you hearing the voice of a teacher or a parent? When does it come? How does it make you feel? Would you say the same thing to someone else?

- Finally, convert your investigation into intention. Decide to change the thought pattern – as soon as the thought comes, let it go.

Then things can start to change. Going through this process with some-one else, such as a friend or a counsellor, can be helpful.

Emotional release

Emotional release is not something you can teach a student; rather it just tends to happen to students as they practise yoga. It can be very confusing for people to leave a yoga class in tears or feeling angry and depressed or paranoid for no apparent reason, so as a teacher it is important for you to explain that this bubbling over of emotion is something that often happens and is a positive, important part of the process, and to help your students to deal with it when it happens.

- During a yoga practice we work on the physical body. That is obvious. But we also work on our subtle bodies, the body of energy and the bodies of emotions and mind. Just as we unlock blockages and stored tensions in the physical body, we unlock blockages and old patterns on the emotional and mental level. Sometimes old events that have had a strong emotional impact on us get stored unconsciously. These old events affect our responses and sometimes cause us to repeatedly act out our patterns of behaviour.
- A yoga practice can unblock these patterns. Releasing physical blockages can feel uncomfortable as toxins are released. In a similar way, releasing emotional blockages can feel uncomfortable as we re-experience toxic emotions.

If a student leaves a yoga class feeling angry or depressed or vulnerable for no apparent reason, it may be because they are releasing blockages on the mental or emotional level. While this is going on, the important thing for them is not to react to the emotion. Advise the student:

- not to act out the emotion
- to try to hold the emotion and observe it

- to really feel the emotion and experience it
- to accept all emotions without judgement
- to keep going with the practice
- to warn people close to them they are going through a rough patch
- to be very gentle with themselves
- to seek other therapies to help them deal with especially difficult emotions

My experience is that these emotionally intense periods normally pass in a few months at the most, but are rarely cleared up completely in one go. We are all very complex and we tend to store deep-seated emotional issues in layers that we access slowly as we develop.

HAPPINESS

For me there is no point in adopting a practice that does not increase happiness, be it a spiritual practice or otherwise. Happiness may not always be experienced in the short term: anything that is truly transformational is bound to include uncomfortable and challenging periods. But ultimately the practice is about increasing happiness and decreasing suffering. Talking about happiness in a yoga class is a safe and neutral way to bring up the spiritual aspects of yoga. Yoga's version of 'happiness' may differ from the idea as we conceive it. In yoga the concept of happiness is not a euphoric reaction to a positive event, it is more like our idea of contentment. In yogic philosophy, if we can get to a state where the highs and lows of life do not pull us emotionally up and down, but instead find a place of balance and contentment, that is seen as happiness.

TEACHING HAPPINESS

I am not suggesting that I have an easy formula to teach people to be happy, but maybe as teachers we can suggest ways that yoga can play its part.

Happiness through focus

When we are doing something that fully engages our attention and awareness, then we are more likely to be happy. Sometimes this absorption just happens, but it is also something we can actively work on. If we become tired, distracted or bored during a yoga practice, we can move past these feelings by focusing on our breath. By tuning in, feeling the temperature and texture of the air, feeling the movement of our lungs and chest, we can move past that feeling of tiredness or distraction to a state of absorption and happiness.

It would be an amazing thing to live our whole lives in such a state. If we learn to achieve it during our yoga practice, we can start to apply it to the rest of our lives. We can also note which activities in our lives foster that feeling and try to do them more often.[41]

Happiness through clarity

As described above, yoga can help us to become aware of our patterns of behaviour and unconscious assumptions. This can help us see our selves and the world more clearly. When we can see with greater clarity, we can react more honestly and can consequently become happier.

Happiness through the breath

A yoga practice has a profound effect on the body and mind. One way this works is through the breath via the nervous system. The nervous system is an ancient biological network of information. It is responsible for controlling biological processes and movement within the body. It receives information, interprets it and causes the body to react. The parasympathetic nervous system is activated when there is no danger perceived by the body. This is the part of the nervous system that calms and relaxes the body (see Chapter 2 for a fuller explanation). It brings the heart rate and blood pressure down to normal and reduces muscle tension.

Explain to your students that a yoga practice affects the mind as well as the body, that when you breathe slowly and deeply, keeping the eyes still and the face relaxed, this signals to the body/mind that there is no danger, and activates the parasympathetic nervous system. We feel relaxed and at ease and connected to people around us. We feel happy.

YOGIC CONCEPTS: THE YAMAS

Dating from around 2,000 years ago, Patañjali's Yoga Sutras are often considered to be the most important of the yogic texts and as a yoga teacher you should be familiar with them. They state very clearly one idea of what yoga is, and how yoga can help address problems in the human condition that are common to us all.

Patañjali describes yoga as an eightfold path (confusingly also called 'ashtanga', which actually means eight limbs). These eight 'limbs' are:

- yamas (attitude to other people; see below)
- niyamas (personal observances; see Chapter 7)
- asana (physical poses)
- pranayama (breathing exercises)
- pratyahara (withdrawal of the senses or the ability not to get distracted by what is going on around you)
- dharana (ability to concentrate)
- dhyana (true meditation)
- samadhi (a state of bliss)

The first of these 'limbs', the yamas, consists of five ethical principles, suggestions for how to interact with the world around us. These are:

- ahimsa (non-violence)
- satya (truthfulness)
- asteya (not stealing)
- brahmacharya (using sexual energy wisely)
- aparigraha (non-grasping)

Talking about the yamas is a very good way of introducing yoga's spiritual aspect into a class. As a teacher it is important that you think about these concepts before you talk about them to a class. Choose one each month and try to live with the idea in your mind. You might try keeping a journal of what issues come up for you as you focus on one particular yama. Read different translations of the Yoga Sutras and think about other people's interpretations.

Also think about why we are asked to follow the yamas. Do we need to be 'good people' to be spiritual? In modern society and many religions, one is 'encouraged' to follow certain rules out of fear of punishment. In the yoga tradition it does not work in quite the same way. The idea is more that by living an ethical life we will become happier, healthier, calmer and more able to gain peace and clarity. Studies have shown that living life with feelings of hatred, anger and selfishness makes us unhappy and increases all indicators of stress. There is also evidence to suggest that stress and unhappiness make us more likely to die prematurely.[42] It makes sense to act ethically, even from a purely selfish point of view, since this makes us happier and healthier.

TEACHING THE YAMAS

When we are practising Ashtanga, we often come up against big issues: how we deal with obstacles, how we react when things are difficult for us (or when they are easy), how we feel about ourselves and others. This means that we can often see clearly our relationship to the yamas through our asana practice and then understand patterns that occur in the rest of our lives, and this makes Ashtanga a particularly good vehicle for teaching the yamas.

Living with the yamas applies the ideals of yoga to the whole of our lives, not just to the body and mind in a yoga class. What we do for an hour a week during our yoga class is important, but what we do during our whole lives is far more important. It can be easy to feel the peace and stillness when we are in our yoga class, but can we feel it in the rest of our lives as well?

It is important that you explain to your students that in the yoga texts there are often lists of suggestions for how to live your life. Explain that these lists are not commands, but ways of living that can help you become happier and more peaceful. Unhelpful traits such as untruthfulness or acquisitiveness are likely to create a degree of mental stress and disquiet that will make it hard to develop the stillness and peace needed for spiritual development.

Some of the yamas are easier to talk about than others. I find the ones that can be related directly to an asana practice are the most accessible: ahimsa (non-violence), satya (truthfulness) and aparigraha (non-grasping).

Ahimsa

Ahimsa is defined as 'not causing injury to anyone, including animals, in any form, at any time, for any reason, in word, thought or deed'.[43]

- When working with this concept, it is important to start with the self. Before we think about whether we are non-violent towards others, we have to ask whether we are non-violent towards ourselves.
- When teaching, explain that ahimsa can be considered the most important yama, and that we should start by thinking about how we treat ourselves.

- Illustrate to your students that it is relatively easy to see whether we are non-violent to ourselves in thought, word and deed while we are on the yoga mat:
  - o Do we push ourselves so hard that it hurts?
  - o Do we allow ourselves to rest when we really need to?
  - o Do we criticise ourselves when we find things hard?
  - o Do we treat ourselves with respect and love?
- We are often hard on ourselves. Ask your students to notice what they say to themselves. If they judge and criticise themselves, then they probably do it to other people, too.
- Then the next stage is to notice how ahimsa applies to the rest of our lives:
  - o Do we cause harm in the ways we react to people around us? (Remember: in thought as well as in word and deed.)
  - o How do we treat the environment and animals?

Satya

Satya is 'truthfulness in thought, word or deed'.[43]

- When talking about truthfulness, the starting point is once again how truthful we are to ourselves in our asana practice:
  - o Are we pushing and pulling ourselves further into an asana in a way that is not right for our bodies?
  - o Are we putting up with unhealthy pain in order to get into a pose?
- In daily life we can observe ourselves in conversations: when we decide to say something, is it true? Why do we want to say it?
- The process of working through our learned, unthinking patterns in this way will help us see things more clearly, react to situations consciously and therefore live in a more truthful way.

In his book *Yoga Mala*, the guru of Ashtanga yoga Sri K. Pattabhi Jois says that 'truth must be pleasant to others'. Sometimes the truth hurts, and in these situations non-violence may take precedence over truthfulness. It is interesting to think about the times when ahimsa and satya come into conflict in your life. What do you do? And why? Perhaps sometimes we even use truthfulness as an excuse to hurt someone intentionally. Think about the balance between compassion and truthfulness.

Aparigraha

Aparigraha is defined as 'only taking as much food as we need... and not desiring things of enjoyment which are superfluous to the physical body'.[44] This concept is often simplified as 'non-grasping'.

- In applying aparigraha to a yoga practice, notice when you feel competitive:
  o Do you want to be able to do what other people can do?
  o Are you jealous and resentful of other people who are strong and flexible and able to do asana more easily or more beautifully than you?
- Jealousy and resentment are very difficult emotions to live with. When teaching asana it is important to stress to students that there is no such thing as a perfect asana, that everybody is different, and that what is 'perfect' will be different for different people.
- Rather than conceptualising an asana as a challenge to put your body in a certain shape, see the asana as a way of exploring your body.
- Try to appreciate what your body can do right now, feel it getting stronger and more flexible, and enjoy the process.
- We might want to be able to touch our toes, or jump through, or get the next posture, but as soon as we achieve that goal, more than likely we will want something else. This pattern can carry on for years, always making us dissatisfied with our practice and ourselves. For our own peace of mind, it is good to step out of that loop and start appreciating how lucky we are to be practising asana at all. How lucky we are to have healthy bodies and the resources that allow us to practise yoga.

The way of working with all these behavioural patterns is first of all to notice what our pattern is, to observe it – not to judge it – and then have the intention to change it.

YOGA AS ENERGY: HATHA YOGA

The Yoga Sutras are part of the classical yoga tradition and were written around 2,000 years ago. Hatha yoga is a more recent tradition dating from around 500 years ago. Its key text is the Hatha Yoga Pradipika – as with the Yoga Sutras, you should be familiar with the ideas it presents. Hatha yoga places particular emphasis on using the body to affect our energetic body for spiritual purposes.

HATHA YOGA AND ASHTANGA YOGA

There is often a distinction made between 'yoga' on the one hand, and 'meditation' on the other, with the idea that meditation is somehow more spiritual, and that we do yoga (or asana) just in order to be able to sit comfortably to meditate. There is a prevalent idea that the physical is separate from the spiritual.

However, in Ashtanga yoga, as well as in tantric yoga traditions, the relationship between the physical and the spiritual is more complex. The body is seen as the primary vehicle for spiritual development. One of the ideas from this strand of yogic philosophy is that practices we do in an Ashtanga yoga class such as asana (physical poses), pranayama (breathing), bandha (engaging certain muscles within the body), chanting and mudra (gestures with the body) all work on the energetic body as well as the physical.

This belief that working on the energetic body is in itself a spiritual process derives from the hatha yoga tradition. According to hatha yoga, we have a total of five bodies all inhabiting roughly the same physical space. An asana practice will affect all five: the physical body (annamaya kosha), the energetic body (pranamaya kosha), the mental body (manomaya kosha), the emotional body (vijnanamaya kosha), and the bliss body (anandamaya kosha).[45]

The effects of yoga practice on the physical body are the most obvious – for example, the stretching of muscles and connective tissue. The effects on the other bodies are just as strong but often less apparent.

TEACHING YOGA AS ENERGY

Pranamaya kosha and kundalini

- Explain at the beginning of a class that in esoteric yogic theory we have three main lines of energy (or 'nadis') in the body: the pingala (dynamic, sun energy), the ida (passive, moon energy) and the sushumna.

- According to hatha yoga the idea of practising asana and pranayama is to purify the body and lines of energy so that our kundalini energy (which is symbolised as a serpent sleeping at the base of the spine) wakes up and travels up the sushumna and out the top of the head, leading to a state of bliss and awakening.
- You could then go on to talk about nadis, mudras and bandhas to help students sense and access this energy.

Nadis

- At the beginning of the class, suggest that the students focus on five lines of energy in the body.
- They all start just below the navel and radiate outwards: two down the legs, two up the spine and down the arms and one up the spine and out the top of the head.
- At various points throughout the practice, ask your students if they can become aware of the energy flows. Trikonasana is particularly good for this.[46]
- Explain that yoga does not affect only our physical bodies, but also affects our flows of energy.
- Explain that these flows are similar to meridians in the Chinese system and that in the yogic system they are called nadis.

Mudras and bandhas

- Explain that when we place our bodies in certain positions, called mudras, we are affecting the way the energy flows.
- When we place our hands together in prayer position, or hook the first two fingers around the big toes or place our thumb and first finger together for the breathing at the end of the Ashtanga yoga sequence, we are working on our energetic body.
- Mention to students that the effects on the energetic body can be felt as buzzing or vibration. After the sun salutations, stop the class in Tadasana and suggest they focus on the sensations

they feel in the palms of the hands. There is often a fairly clear sensation of buzzing or tingling.

- During the breathing at the end, suggest that students focus on the place where the thumb and finger meet in chin mudra and see if they can feel any sensations there.
- Explain that the bandhas, as well as being physical locks, are energetic locks aimed at increasing energy in the body and redirecting its flow (just like mudras).
- Try teaching a whole class just focused on engaging the bandhas (see Chapter 3, Teaching the Bandhas). By the end of the class there is normally a clear feeling of lightness and ease in the postures that usually is not there.

SUMMARY

It is important to talk about the spiritual aspects of yoga, even if only during some classes, and even if only in small doses. It is equally important not to preach. People generally find the spiritual aspects of yoga more accessible or palatable when you mention more neutral concepts such as clarity, focus, happiness, peace and well-being. What we mean by the spiritual aspect is normally very personal, and normally evolves over time as our understanding changes.

Not everyone will agree with your view of spirituality, and that is fine. But if talking about it in your yoga class makes your students think and helps them to clarify what they think, then that can only be a good thing. Start small with something you are confident about and see how that goes and how it develops.

SUGGESTED READING

My first suggestion is to read the Yoga Sutras, and to read as many translations as you can. I especially like *Four Chapters on Freedom* by Swami Satyananda (Yoga Publications Trust, Bihar, India, 2005) and *How to Know God: The Yoga Aphorisms of Patañjali* by Christopher Isherwood and Swami Prabhavananda (Vedanta Press, 1953).

For the ideas of hatha yoga and tantric ideas of energy, read the *Hatha Yoga Pradipika*. I have found the most helpful translation to be by Swami

Muktibodhananda (Yoga Publications, 1985). Also very clear and informative is *Prana Pranayama Prana Vidya* by Swami Niranjanananda Saraswati (Yoga Publications, 1994).

For general ideas of yoga and spirituality, I recommend *Yoga and the Quest for the True Self* by Stephen Cope (Bantam Books, 1999) and *Yoga: The Spirit and Practice of Moving into Stillness* by Eric Schiffmann (Pocket Books, 1996).

For explanations and ideas for living with the yamas there is the excellent *Mindful Yoga Mindful Life: A Guide for Everyday Practice* by Charlotte Bell (Rodmell Press, 2007). This book was very inspiring and helpful to me when writing this chapter.

CHAPTER 7
TEACHING YOGA

ETHICS FOR YOGA TEACHERS

In this chapter I set out suggestions for ethical yoga teaching with particular reference to Patañjali's yamas and niyamas from the Yoga Sutras. These ethical guidelines can help you to teach and relate to students in a way that is clear and strong. All teacher–pupil relationships are complicated and the relationship between a yoga teacher and student can be especially intense. I have seen situations develop between teachers and students that are awkward and unhelpful. In almost all cases the situation would have been avoided if the teacher had acted in accordance with the yamas and niyamas. It is very easy to make statements like this with hindsight, and no one is perfect, but your students' experience and your job as a teacher will be more productive and more enjoyable if you follow these principles.

YAMAS AND NIYAMAS

In the previous chapter, we looked at the yamas, one of the eight 'limbs' of the Yoga Sutras, and saw how they can guide all yoga practitioners in their quest for spiritual development. In this chapter, we will revisit the yamas, but this time learn how they can form the basis for a healthy, productive relationship between teacher and students. We will also examine another of the 'limbs', the niyamas, which contain much valuable ethical insight. As well as benefiting us, observing the yamas and niyamas will benefit those around us.

THE YAMAS

As we have seen, the yamas are five principles that help us act towards the people around us in a way that is helpful for our spiritual development (sometimes called external disciplines). The five yamas are:

Ahimsa (non-violence): This is a commitment to live a life without causing harm to our selves or to others around us. This applies mentally as well as physically. It is often considered to be the most important yama. More than living without harming, ahimsa implies living with compassion and love.

Satya (truthfulness): Satya is one of the most complicated of the yamas. In most circumstances telling the truth is clearly the right thing to do. However, sometimes satya comes into conflict with ahimsa – truthfulness can be harmful. When communicating with other people, we need to consider not only what is truthful but also what is compassionate, helpful and loving.

Asteya (not stealing): As well as literally not stealing, asteya can be interpreted in a wider sense. Do we take more than our share? Do we take others' time? Do we feel as if we have enough or do we want to take more?

Brahmacharya (celibacy): This is one of the difficult yamas to translate in a way that is true to the original intention and relevant to a modern yoga teacher and student. Rather than sexual abstinence, a more helpful interpretation might be honesty, compassion and integrity in our sexual relationships.

Aparigraha (not grasping): Modern society often makes people feel they have to acquire things or live in a certain way in order to be happy. This feeling can stop us from enjoying our life and ultimately stop us from being free. The yearning for what we don't have and the fear of losing what we do have are a huge barrier to contentment and flowing with life.

THE NIYAMAS

The niyamas are five principles for how we can act within ourselves to help our yoga practice (sometimes called internal disciplines). The five niyamas are:

Shaucha (purity): Purity can apply to your body, your environment, your diet, your mind – in fact, to all aspects of your life. Living in a pure way can make your life lighter and clearer and more beautiful.

Santosha (contentment): This is being satisfied with, and accepting of, our life and circumstance. It is not happiness. It is being balanced and grounded in our selves.

Tapas (fire of transformation): In order to grow and evolve in our spiritual life, we need to practise and sometimes to practise hard. Most growth or change that is worthwhile will not be easy to achieve. We need to have been through the 'fire of transformation' to be able to help our students make the same journey.

Swadhyaya (self-study): This applies to external and internal study. We will become better, more rounded yoga teachers if we read what others have written, attend workshops, talk to other teachers and students and all the time learn, learn, learn. Even if we learn how not to do something, that is still a valuable lesson. Equally, we will evolve if we always strive to learn about our selves. What are our patterns? Who pushes our buttons and why? How can we become the best we can be?

Ishvarapranidhana (devotion to God): This is another aspect of the Yoga Sutras that is difficult to present in a way that is relevant and helpful to a modern audience. It might have more resonance if 'God' is replaced by 'spiritual transformation' or 'the good of all'. However you phrase it, the important idea is that we work and strive not just for ourselves but for something bigger.

CREATING A SAFE LEARNING ENVIRONMENT

Often students will have periods when they feel vulnerable and sensitive as they progress with their yoga practice. It is part of your job to create a safe space for students to go through their process of transformation. This means that you need to be calm, consistent, trustworthy and caring. Also aim to cultivate these traits among your students, so everyone in the class helps to build a positive environment.

There may be times when a student will break down crying or become angry and frustrated or be attention-seeking or critical – you need to be able to accommodate this without losing your own centre. Allow them the space to express what they feel, comfort them and reassure them if necessary. If they are angry or critical you may feel the need to put your own point of view across, but try to do this calmly without anger or recrimination.

If you are faced with a situation relating to a particular student and you are unsure what to do, it can be very useful to use the yamas and niyamas as a guide. Before you take action, ask yourself questions such as:

- Is what I am planning to say or do compassionate?
- Is it truthful?
- Am I acting from jealousy or resentment?
- Would I like to be treated this way myself?
- Am I comfortable telling others about my actions?
- Has this behaviour caused me problems in the past?
- Is this action likely to create suffering?
- If I were another student in the class how would I feel (e.g. if the teacher were giving attention to one student over another)?

Consider consulting a more experienced teacher whom you trust to be your supervisor or mentor or talk things through with your peer group – a group of fellow teachers or friends.[47] However, be sure to respect the confidentiality of the student (see below).

You can tailor this general approach to apply to specific ethical considerations, including the ones below. For each of these areas, I have indicated, where appropriate, which yama or niyama I have drawn upon.

RESPECT

Respect all students regardless of race, gender, sexual orientation, physical ability, financial status or national origin. If you find yourself feeling prejudiced towards a student for whatever reason – perhaps you just find them annoying – observe the emotion and try your best not to act on it. We all have our preconceptions: it is very important to be aware of them and to remember that it is up to us how we act on them. (Ahimsa)

An important part of showing respect to your students is how you present yourself. So, for example:

- Be clean and well presented.
- Dress in a modest manner.
- Avoid misuse of alcohol or drugs while teaching.
- Be mindful of the way you speak – many students will be offended by swearing (religious or otherwise) and it is really unnecessary when you are teaching a yoga class. (Shaucha)

DIFFERENCES OF OPINION

There are often several different ways of approaching each element of a yoga practice and your method is not necessarily the only acceptable one. If a student disagrees with what you are teaching, maybe because a previous teacher taught them differently or maybe due to a physical or emotional block, then you need to respect that. Rather than trying to enforce your point of view, try to turn the situation into a dialogue. Explain the reasons why you think a certain way, then listen to how they see it, and see if you can find a compromise. Ultimately, it is up to the student to decide what they want to do – it is their body and their practice. If it is something you feel very strongly about, you may have to suggest they find another teacher. Approaching situations lightly and with humour can often help a student accept teaching they may find difficult, but judge this on an individual basis.

FEEDBACK

When you observe a student in difficulty with a particular aspect of their practice, give feedback in a positive, constructive way. Focus not on what they are doing wrong, but on what they need to do to put it right. Give adjustments with gentleness and compassion (see Chapter 11, Adjustments). (Ahimsa)

CONFIDENTIALITY

Confidentiality should always be respected. If a student tells you something personal, do not repeat it to other students or teachers. Sometimes you may want to ask advice from a senior teacher or peer about a student, which would mean breaking confidentiality. If this is the case, protect the student's identity if this is possible and, if not, ask the other teacher to respect confidentiality. (Satya)

SEX AND RELATIONSHIPS

This can be a problematic area. One thing is clear: as a yoga teacher you should not use your classes as a place to search for potential sexual partners. This would set up completely the wrong atmosphere for a yoga class.

Some people would say that a teacher should absolutely never have a sexual relationship with a student. However, to me this seems too rigid. I think it is possible for two people to meet as equals and have a happy relationship as yoga teacher and student. I know of several successful couples who met in this way. For it to work, you would have to avoid your personal relationship with your partner affecting your teacher–student relationship and try not to allow it to affect the rest of the yoga class. This means that you need to be able to give your partner clear, relevant unbiased instruction and relate to them in a way that does not draw attention or cause embarrassment or resentment in the rest of the class. This would require a fair amount of skilful negotiation, but I think it is possible. You would also have to ask yourself whether you believe that you and the student could deal with the potential pitfalls, including how you would handle it if the relationship ended unhappily. If you were unsure, the safest course of action might be for your partner to switch to another yoga class.

Be aware of the balance of power in the relationship between you and your students. Some students may be vulnerable or impressionable and may become attracted to you simply because you are 'the yoga teacher'. If you encounter situations like this, help the student to cultivate a more balanced, less idealised picture of you. This could be a positive foundation for a supportive friendship with a vulnerable person. Or you may feel that it is better to back off and not pursue a friendship with them. Certainly, you should not have a sexual relationship with anyone who is vulnerable.

Personally, I have been in a monogamous relationship all the time I have been a yoga teacher, so I can't speak from direct experience. My husband has been my student for over ten years and this has worked very well for us, but we did not meet through yoga.

This is a difficult area and you need to think very seriously about your role as a teacher if you are going to start a relationship with a student. Consulting your mentor or peer group might help you to see the full picture. (Brahmacharya)

AUTHENTICITY

Your teaching will be far more effective if you teach from the heart and are true to yourself. Bear in mind the following points.

- A yoga teacher is always learning: from their own practice, from their students, from books and other teachers, from thoughts and from opening themselves to inspiration. (Swadhyaya)

- Walk your talk. If you teach something in the class, aspire to live it in the whole of your life. At the same time, do not try to appear perfect or to represent yourself as something you are not. (Satya)

- Always represent your education, training and experience accurately to employers and students and only teach what you know from experience and practice. Reading about something from a book or repeating something from another teacher is not a substitute for your own knowledge. (Satya)

- If teaching a student is beyond your ability, then refer them to a teacher who can help them. For example, if a student has mental health or addiction problems that you are not qualified to deal with, refer them to a class specifically for people with those problems. Likewise, if a student has a more advanced practice than you, refer them to a more senior teacher. (Satya)

- A yoga teacher should have their own regular yoga practice, and a constant commitment to continued learning. (Tapas)

- Embrace yoga as a way of life. Your students will look to you as an example of what yoga will give them in their life. Do you stand up to their scrutiny? (Tapas)

- Try to encourage your students not to be dependent on you. Encourage them to rely on themselves. (Aparigraha)

- Trust in your knowledge and ability to teach, share what you know and enjoy what you do. If you are not happy in what you are teaching it is unlikely your students will be happy. (Santosha)

- Strive to become the best you can be, in order to help your students. Do this for the good of all and for the joy of doing your best, not to feed your ego and become rich and famous. (Ishvarapranidhana)

MONEY AND THE HARD SELL

As yoga teachers, we are often self-employed and money and finances can be a difficult issue. It is important to value yourself and your skills, but at the same time to be fair and reasonable in your financial dealings. Make sure you allow yourself time off and do not take on so many classes that you are too tired to give your best in each class. (Aparigraha)

It is fairly common for teachers to encourage students to sign up for workshops, buy yoga mats or yoga clothes or go on yoga holidays. There is a balance to be struck between letting your students know what you have to offer, and giving them a hard sell while they are in their post-yoga glow. (Ahimsa)

ACKNOWLEDGING OTHERS

Credit your teachers where appropriate. If you are passing on a piece of knowledge you learned from a particular teacher, it is good practice to name them and credit their teaching. Equally, it is important not to use your class as a platform to criticise other yoga teachers or schools. You should also give credit to students for their progress or transformation – you may have helped, but the student ultimately was the one who did the work. (Asteya/Ahimsa)

If you experience jealousy or resentment in relation to a student's progress, then observe this emotion and work with it as part of your yoga practice, but try not to act on it in relation to that student. (Aparigraha)

SUMMARY

No one is perfect and no one expects you to be. All anyone can do is their best. If you make a mistake, the important thing is to admit it, rectify any damage you have done, learn from it, and then move on. Dwelling on something and feeling guilty does not help anyone. Talk to other yoga teachers, share your experiences and ask them how they have handled similar situations.

SUGGESTED READING

Donna Farhi's excellent *Teaching Yoga: Exploring the Teacher–Student Relationship* (Rodmell Press, 2006) was very helpful to me in writing this section. I also especially like her interpretation of the yamas and niyamas in *Yoga Mind, Body & Spirit: A Return to Wholeness* (Henry Holt, 2000).

CHAPTER 8
TEACHING YOGA

TEACHING POINTS

Refining your verbal cues so that you communicate effectively is an ongoing process for any teacher. If students are always getting things wrong, it is your responsibility to communicate effectively so they get it right. Teaching points need to be clear, concise and unambiguous. This is especially true if you are teaching a led class where the breath is counted. You will have minimal time to make the point and practically no time to correct any misunderstandings.

In this chapter I give general guidelines for how to formulate your teaching points, followed by general teaching points for the breath, feet, legs, focus and awareness and relaxing. In the main part of the chapter are my suggestions for teaching points for each asana. They are all tried-and-tested phrases that are succinct and clear, and that I have found to be effective. They are not necessarily complete grammatical sentences, but short phrases that describe exactly what a student should try to do with an asana. Obviously this list is not exhaustive and is offered as inspiration in helping you find your own voice as a teacher.

WHAT TO SAY

Before we focus on teaching points for the individual asana, bear in mind these important general principles.

Positive: Phrase your instructions in the positive. Say, 'soften the shoulders' rather than 'don't tense the shoulders'.

Inclusive: When giving directions, always imagine how your less able students will react to them. For example, say 'sink the heels towards the floor' rather than 'sink the heels to the floor'. This way, people will not feel they are 'doing it wrong' if they can't reach their heels all the way down. Similarly, if you are giving different options, give the easiest option first. If you go from difficult to easy, it can make people taking the easier option feel inadequate.

Logical: Work your way logically around the body. For standing postures, start at the foundation – the feet – and work your way up. Alternatively, you may start at the core and work your way out. If you dot around the body, it can be confusing to students.

Sparing: Do not give too many instructions. Two or three is enough for each posture. Allow the students space.

Relevant: Look at what the students are doing so you can make the points relevant – and make sure the general instructions you give to the whole class are relevant to all body types. Do not simply rattle off teaching points for the sake of it. It is important to allow the students some silence. You do not have to be giving instructions all the time. Silence allows the students time for their own experience.

Consistent: When teaching a led class, the order of instructions should always be: breath, instruction, teaching point. For example, at the beginning of the sun salutation:

> Breath – 'inhale'
> Instruction – 'reach up'
> Teaching point – 'soften the shoulders'

Keep this order consistent throughout the class.

Natural: When you become more experienced, do not plan everything you are going to say in advance. Try to get your thinking mind out of the way and allow inspiration to come to you.

GENERAL TEACHING POINTS

BREATH

- Ujjayi breath
- Slow, deep breath
- Breathe into the ribcage, into the chest
- Soften the breath
- Flow with your breath
- Create space on the inhalation
- Relax/move into the space on the exhalation
- Listen to your breath
- Full, deep inhalation [especially for postures such as up-dog when the breath tends to be shortened]
- Full, deep exhalation [especially for Chatturanga Dandasana when the breath tends to be shortened]

FEET

- Even balance between the heels and balls of the feet
- Relax the toes
- Lift up the inner edge of the foot
- Press down the outer edge of the foot
- Sink the feet down into the ground and feel an opposite energy lifting you up [standing postures]
- Lengthen the feet [especially in down-dog]
- Press feet gently away from each other [standing postures]
- Flex the feet/toes point up towards the ceiling [sitting postures]
- Extend the heels to lengthen the calves and activate the legs

LEGS

- Energise the legs
- Pull up on the front thighs
- Keep the legs straight but the knees slightly soft

FOCUS AND AWARENESS

- Notice where your attention is
- Listen to the sound of your breath
- Feel your foundation in your feet

RELAXING

Middle path: Often students come to yoga with an attitude of striving too hard; this is counterproductive. It is in the breath and the softening that transformation of mind and body takes place. Forcing the body to stretch might make muscles longer, but learning to listen to your breath and your body, and learning to connect to your inner stillness and peace is truly transformative. Your job will often be to encourage people to back off and stop trying so hard. Sometimes pushing too hard will just cause the body to tense up. To simplify, there are two general patterns: trying too hard and taking it too easy. It is worth talking about these two patterns in class and suggesting that if a student recognises themselves in one or the other they should observe their pattern and try to find a balanced middle ground where they try, but not too hard (see Chapter 6).

Tension: Students often have habits of tensing muscles they do not actually need. Most commonly these will be in the jaw and the shoulders. This paradoxically creates tension in the body instead of getting rid of it.

Pain: It is important to explain to beginners that practising yoga should not hurt. A lot of people are stuck in the 'no pain no gain' mind set, which is inapplicable to yoga. If the body is in pain it is more likely to tense up than stretch out. A gentle stretch is what we are looking for; we go to the edge and then relax and breathe and explore the edge. Very intense sensations, especially sharp pains in the joints, especially the knees and the spine, are definitely neither productive nor safe. (See 'Signals to stop stretching the body' in Chapter 5, Injuries.)

You need to translate these relatively complex ideas into simple, easily digestible teaching points such as the following:

- If it hurts or you cannot breathe, then back off
- Soften the body within the posture
- Relax your face

- Relax the shoulders
- Maintain a sense of fluidity within the posture (we are over 60 per cent water)
- Enjoy what your body can do right now
- Accept what your body can do right now
- Tune in to how your body feels right in this moment
- Use the asana as an opportunity to explore your body
- Approach each asana with curiosity: what will my body do today?

ASANA TEACHING POINTS

I have given instructions for the first (right) side of each posture. Most of these teaching points are positive instructions, some are 'watch out' points.

SAMASTITIHI

It is important to set Samastitihi before you start the first sun salutation and periodically throughout the class. This will put the body in a neutral position at the beginning of the class and wipe the slate clean in between postures. It allows beginners to have a rest and gives the whole class a chance to tune in to their bodies.

- Tune in to how your body feels right now
- Can you feel your heart beat?
- What sensations do you feel in the palms of your hands?

Samastitihi helps students to start to develop sensitivity to their body and breath. Stop the class every now and then and have students stand with their eyes closed and focus on their body and the breath in Samastitihi. It does break the flow and is not traditional, but it is a useful way to focus awareness.

For Samastitihi, always say the same things in the same order – it helps students to remember the points and it sets the mind and body into yoga mode.

- Feet together
- Toe bones touching
- Ankle bones as close as comfortable
- Spread the toes
- Relax the toes

- Even balance between front and back of feet
- Lift inner arches of feet
- Engage the front of the thighs
- Moola bandha, uddiyana bandha
- Shoulders relaxing back and down
- Head straight on your neck
- Back of the neck long
- See straight in front of you
- Ujjayi breathing

SUN SALUTATIONS

Inhale

Urdhva Vrksasana (reach up):

- Soften the shoulders

In this initial movement students often over-reach and end up hunching up the shoulders and also over-arching the lower back. The instruction to soften the shoulders can be given generally to the whole class, but if a student is over-arching the lower back, speak to them individually and explain to them that this creates tension in the hips and can put pressure on the spine.

Exhale

Uttanasana A (fold down):

- Draw the navel in
- Relax the head and the neck

Inhale

Uttanasana B (lift the chest):

- Broaden the collar bones
- Back of the neck long
- Lengthen the spine
- Lengthen the front of the body
- Look to the third eye

Exhale

Chatturanga Dandasana:

- Not too low with the shoulders [if the shoulders are lowered too near to the floor, this will hunch the whole shoulder joint and create tension in the trapezius muscle – a student should only lower down until the upper arm is parallel to the floor]

- Shoulders away from ears
- Elbows in
- Focus on core strength
- Navel in as you lower
- Engage the front thighs
- Press back into the heels
- Press the elbows back and the chest forwards

Inhale

Urdhva Mukha Svanasana (up-dog):
- Roll the shoulders back and down
- Press down through the hands; press the floor away
- Relax the face
- Lengthen the front of the body
- Breathe up into the chest
- Open the chest
- Broaden across the collar bones
- Relax the muscles in the bum
- Engage the legs
- Engage the front thighs
- Press down through the big toe and the little toe
- Strong moola bandha

Exhale

Adho Mukha Svanasana (down-dog):
- Hands shoulder-width apart
- Fingers spread
- Middle finger points forwards
- Gently press down through the thumb and index finger
- Base of each finger and tip of each finger gently pressing down
- Lower arms rotate in [medial rotation]
- Upper arms rotate out [lateral rotation]
- Armpits rotate towards each other to broaden the shoulders

- Press the floor away from you
- Head moves down towards the floor
- Lift up out of the hands and sink down into the feet
- Relax the head, neck and face
- Lengthen through the sides of the ribcage
- Lengthen from the tailbone to the back of the neck
- The ribcage moves towards the thighs
- Moola bandha, uddiyana bandha
- Engage the front of the thighs
- Rotate the thighs inwards
- Feet hips-width apart
- Spread the toes
- Lift up the inner edge of the feet
- Gently sink the heels towards the floor

Inhale

Virabhadrasana 1:
- Press down with the front heel
- Sink the hips down as you reach up
- Square the hips towards the front
- Square the shoulders towards the front
- Soften the shoulders down

STANDING POSTURES

Padangushtasana/Padahastasana

- Weight even between the heels and balls of the feet [heels and back of the hands for Padahastasana – the gentle pressure on the hands in Padahastasana is a nice counterbalance to all the work the wrists have done in the sun salutations]
- Bend the knees as much as you have to [signals that a student has to bend the knees include: sharp or intense pain; inability to breathe slowly and deeply; desire to clench the teeth and tense the face; and signs that they are not enjoying the practice – also, if you see that a student's back is very curved, they should bend their knees so they can lengthen their spine]

- If the legs are straight – pull up on the front thighs [engaging the quadriceps so the kneecap is drawn up] and rotate the thighs in [medial rotation] to a neutral position
- Strong uddiyana bandha to support the back
- Lengthen through the front of the body, the sides of the ribcage and the core of the spine and the back of the neck
- Relax the head, neck and muscles in the face
- Relax the arms
- Shoulder blades move towards the hips/away from the ears
- Take the knees away from the eyes
- Lengthen the back of the neck
- Belly towards thighs, chest towards the knees, top of the head towards the floor

Utthita Trikonasana

- Neutral position for the hips and spine [students who are either over-arching the lower back or tucking their tailbone too far under need to lengthen the tailbone away from the head to work towards the neutral curves in the back]
- Heels in line
- Lengthen through the sides of the ribcage – especially the side closest to the floor
- Draw the right shoulder away from the right hip
- Lengthen through the spine
- Lengthen from the tailbone to the top of the head
- Keep the back of the neck long
- Rotate the ribcage up towards the ceiling
- Stretch from fingertip to fingertip
- Expand into the posture

Parivrtta Trikonasana

- Distribute the weight evenly through both feet
- Press down with the outer edge of the back foot and the base of the big toe of the front foot

- Both legs straight
- Pull up on the front thighs
- Rotate the thighs in towards each other
- Squeeze the hips together
- Gently nudge the right hip back and in towards the centre line of the body
- Square the hips towards the back
- Rotate from the navel and above
- Use your exhalation and your uddiyana bandha to go into the rotation
- Use resistance between your left hand and the floor to go into the twist
- Top of the head towards the back wall

Utthita Parsvakonasana

- Lift up the inner edge of the back foot
- Press down with the front heel
- Press the feet down and away from each other
- Keep the knee directly above the ankle
- Press the knee back against the arm
- Rest lightly on the hand
- Feel the line of energy from the back foot to the top hand
- Stretch to your fingertips
- Draw the top shoulder down away from the ear
- Back of the neck is long
- Sink the hips down [if a student is very flexible, make sure they do not go too low – thigh parallel to the floor is perfect]
- Right sitting bone in line with the right heel [often students push their bum out behind them and arch the lower back to get down into the posture]
- Rotate the ribcage up to the ceiling
- Top hand above the front foot

Parivrtta Parsvakonasana

- Soften and relax [this is a challenging posture and students often get carried away trying too hard, so emphasise softening in this posture especially]
- Breathe slowly and deeply [again in the intensity of the posture the breath often gets lost]
- Keep the back of the neck long
- Relax the muscles in the face [in their efforts to find their dristi, students often crank the back of the neck and tense the muscles in the forehead]
- Keep length between the feet [students often shuffle their feet closer together as they move between the four triangle asana]
- Press into the back foot
- Lengthen and twist away from the back foot
- Focus on twisting the torso

Prasarita Padottanasana A, B and D

Give the general instructions for the feet and legs (see page 92).

- Toes turned slightly in
- Outside edges of feet parallel
- Lengthen through the spine
- Top of head towards the floor
- Shoulders away from the ears
- Breathe into the ribcage and the chest

Prasarita Padottanasana C

If the arms are far enough over:

- Relax the arms
- Let gravity do the work for you
- Lengthen the arms on the inhalation – relax them on exhalation
- Lengthen the back of the neck
- Create space across the chest and breathe into that space
- Create space across the shoulders

Parsvottanasana

- Body weight even in both feet
- Press down the outer edge of the back foot and the inner edge of the front foot
- Squeeze the hips together
- Hips square to back wall
- Strong uddiyana bandha
- Lengthen the back of the neck
- Draw the shoulders away from the ears
- Shoulders parallel to the floor
- Lift the elbows up towards the ceiling
- Press the hands together

Utthita Hasta Padangushtasana

- Keep the supporting leg straight
- Pull up on the front thigh of the supporting leg
- Right hip comes back and down – level with the left hip
- Right shoulder comes back and down – level with the left shoulder
- Stand a little bit taller
- Keep the gaze point steady
- Strong bandhas
- Relax the shoulders
- Relax the face

When the leg is out to the side:

- Keep the hips central
- Press both hips in towards the central line of the body

Ardha Baddha Padmottanasana

- Supporting leg straight and strong
- Bent leg softens
- Right shoulder relaxes forwards level with the left shoulder
- Relax the head

Utkatasana

- Press the inner thighs together
- Neutral position for the hips
- Soften the front of the ribcage down towards the hips
- Soften the shoulders down
- Lift the face towards the ceiling [it is important not to hang the weight of the head back onto the delicate structure of the neck]
- Back of the neck long
- Sink the hips a little bit lower
- Press the heels into the ground

Virabhadrasana I

See under sun salutation – here you have more time to give ideas:

- Lift up and out of the lower back
- Lengthen the tailbone down towards the floor
- Hips come forwards
- Draw the front of the ribs down towards hips
- Soften the shoulders

Virabhadrasana II

- Press the bent knee back so it is directly above the ankle
- Press down with the heel of the front foot
- Press down the outside edge of the back foot
- Stretch to the fingertips
- Shoulders down
- Chest [sternum] up
- Spine perpendicular to the floor
- Shoulders directly above the hips
- Hips neutral
- Gaze strong and steady

SITTING POSTURES

Dandasana

This posture is like Samastitihi; it is about setting the foundation, finding a neutral position for the spine and wiping the slate clean between other postures.

All these teaching points can apply to all the sitting postures when the legs are straight:

- Flex the feet
- Keep the heels down on the floor (if the heels come off the floor there is a danger of hyper-extension in the knees)
- Press into the heels
- Draw the little toe back level with the big toe
- Engage the front thighs
- Inner thigh moves down towards the floor [medial rotation of thigh]
- Find a central position for the sitting bones – not tipped forwards or backwards
- Keep the bandhas working
- Find a neutral position for the spine
- Find a gentle lift through the spine
- Ground the hands into the floor
- The arms may be straight or bent – shoulders are relaxed and down
- Lengthen the back of the neck
- Look towards the toes

Paschimattanasana

- Draw the navel in as you fold forwards
- Keep the foundation in the legs
- Relax the arms and shoulders
- Draw the shoulder blades down the back towards hips

- Gentle stretch on the back of the legs
- Sitting bones go back and down into the floor
- Lengthen through: the front of the body, back, sides of the ribcage, back of the neck
- Heart towards the feet

Purvattanasana

- Wrists under the shoulders
- Squeeze the feet together
- Squeeze the legs together [squeezing the legs together engages the adductor muscles; these muscles connect the psoas to the rectus abdominus and the pectorals – the strength muscles of the front of the body]
- Press the toes down towards the floor
- Breathe into the chest
- Lift the hips towards the ceiling
- Lift the chest towards the ceiling
- Lift the face towards the ceiling
- Press down through the hands
- Energy in the legs

Ardha Baddha Padma Paschimattanasana

- Engage the straight leg
- Soften the bent leg
- Soften the bent leg down towards the floor
- Soften the right shoulder down towards the floor so the shoulders are parallel to the floor
- Draw the left shoulder back and down so the shoulders are level
- If comfortable in the padmasana, draw the thighs towards each other

Tiriangmukhaikapada Paschimattanasana

- Strongly engage the straight leg and rotate the inner thigh down towards the floor [activating the straight leg is more important in this posture as it keeps the body upright]

- Relax the right hip down towards the floor
- Connect the right toes to the floor
- Press the top of right foot into the floor to encourage the hips towards the ground

Janu Sirsasana A, B and C

- Engage the straight leg
- Relax the bent leg
- Press the right sitting bone back and down
- Rotate the ribcage towards the straight leg
- Lengthen through the sides of the ribcage – especially the left side

Marichyasana A and B

- Keep your foundation in the right foot – as if you are standing on it
- Keep the straight leg active
- Rotate the shoulders level to the floor
- Relax the right sitting bone down towards the floor
- Open the chest

Marichyasana C and D

- Keep your foundation in the right foot – as if you are standing on it
- Both sitting bones move towards the floor
- Keep the straight leg active
- Rotate the shoulders towards the side wall
- Rotation is from the navel and above
- Hips stay level to the front
- Lift through the spine as you twist
- Lengthen upwards on inhalation and twist on exhalation

Navasana

- Squeeze the legs together
- Send energy right to the toes
- Strong bandhas
- Imagine you have a hook to your heart lifting you towards the ceiling
- Draw the shoulder blades down and back
- Send energy to your fingertips
- Lift up out of the lower back

Bhujapidasana

- Keep your foundation in the hands/keep the hands flat down
- Squeeze the feet up towards the body
- Squeeze the legs against arms
- Lift the chest
- Lift the sitting bones
- Lengthen the front of the body

Kurmasana and Supta Kurmasana

- Squeeze the inner thighs against the ribcage [it is best to do this as you enter into the posture]
- Press into the heels
- Broaden across the chest
- Wiggle the shoulders under the calf
- Stay as relaxed as you can
- Keep breathing

Garbha Pindasana

When rolling round:

- Stay as relaxed as you can
- Roll down on the left side of the spine and up on the right
- Exhale down, inhale up

Kukkutasana

- No moola bandha

Baddha Konasana

- Press the heels together
- Relax the knees towards the floor
- Strong uddiyana bandha
- Even stronger moola bandha
- Press the sitting bones back and down
- Relax the shoulders down away from the ears
- Elbows in to the ribcage

Upavishta Konasana

- Keep the legs strongly engaged – to protect the hamstrings
- Keep the knees and feet pointing up towards the ceiling
- Press into the heels
- Keep the foundation in the sitting bones
- Strong bandhas
- Lengthen through the spine and the back of the neck

When balancing:

- Point the toes
- Look up
- Lift the chest

Supta Konasana

- Energy in the legs
- Lift the sitting bones towards the ceiling

Supta Padangushtasana

- Left leg moves down towards the floor

- Use the left hand to encourage the left leg down
- Point the left foot
- Sitting bones move towards the floor
- Right sitting bone moves in towards the centre line of the body
- Lift the chin to the shin or chest towards the knee
- Use the bandhas

When the leg is out to the side:

- Keep the left side of the hips down on the floor
- Relax both shoulders down towards the floor
- Bring the right heel down towards the floor
- Turn your head to look directly to the side

Ubhaya Padangushtasana

- Straighten the spine to catch the balance
- Point the feet
- Lift up out of the lower back
- Lift the chest up to the ceiling
- Draw the shoulder blades down and back

Urdhva Mukha Paschimattanasana

Same as for Ubhaya Padangushtasana

Setu Bandhasana

- Press the feet into the floor
- Work towards straightening the legs
- Lift the chest
- Nasagrai dristi – look to your nose [it often feels strange to a student to look to their nose in back bends; the natural instinct seems to be to look up. The nasagrai dristi is an energetic counterbalance to discourage throwing back the head]

FINISHING POSTURES

Urdhva Dhanurasana

- Lengthen the front of the body
- Breathe into the front of the body
- Work towards straightening the arms, then work on straightening the legs
- Soften the muscles in the bottom
- Engage the muscles in the legs
- Squeeze the inner thighs towards each other
- Stay grounded in the feet

From this point on, I think it is good to give more silence in the class – allow students to calm down and go inwards.

Salamba Sarvangasana

- Energy in the legs
- Energy in the feet
- Lift through the inner thighs
- Think about this pose in terms of being Tadasana upside-down
- Soften breath
- Look towards the navel
- Gently squeeze the legs together
- Point the toes
- Fingers point up to the ceiling
- Elbows move towards each other
- Make sure there is space between the back of the neck and the floor
- Keep a sense of space between the chin and the chest

Halasana

- Keep the legs active
- Lift the sitting bones up
- Lengthen through the arms

- Top of the feet flat on the floor
- Lift the thighs
- Stay light on the toes

Karnapidasana

- Release moola bandha
- Bring the knees towards the ears
- If the feet are still off the floor then keep the hands on the back
- If the knees are by the ears then gently press the ears with the knees
- Feet stay together

Urdhva Padmasana

- Engage both bandhas

Pindasana

- See if you can bring the knees closer together

Matsyasana

- Arch the chest up towards the ceiling
- Lengthen through the spine
- Lift out of the lower back
- Sink the knees towards the floor

Uttana Padasana

- Nasagri dristi
- Keep the lift in the chest
- Squeeze the inner thighs together
- Strong bandhas

Sirsasana

- Press down with the forearms and the side of the wrists
- Elbows squeeze towards each other

- Lift the shoulders away from the floor
- Press the shoulder blades against the back
- Draw the shoulder blades towards the hips
- Draw the shoulder blades away from each other
- Keep the front of the ribcage coming towards the spine
- Keep the weight even on both arms
- Relax the fingers
- Use the strength in the arms to take pressure off the top of the head
- Try to have a slight space between the top of the head and the floor
- Strong bandhas
- Pubic bone forwards – heels back
- Energy in the legs
- Energy in the feet
- Press up into the feet
- Lift through the inner legs to the big-toe joint
- Squeeze the legs together
- Lift the legs up out of the hips
- Lift the hips away from the shoulders
- Lift the shoulders away from the floor

Shavasana

- Relax the breath – normal breathing
- Allow the head and body to become heavy and sink down into the floor
- Allow your thoughts to drift through your mind
- Completely relax, completely let go
- If the lower back is uncomfortable, bend your knees up and place your feet flat on the floor

TEACHING THE SANSKRIT COUNT

The Sanskrit count is both lovely to teach and lovely to hear while practising. It gives a beautiful rhythm to the class. Do not worry too much about being completely correct at first – just do it, enjoy it and work towards getting it right over time.

This chapter is intended as a beginner's guide for new teachers to start teaching with a count. It does not give detailed instructions on how to get students into postures – knowledge of the postures and the sequence is assumed. The main objective of this guide is to keep the class flowing together. This means that the students all go into and come out of asana together. The more the class moves together, the clearer the focus for everyone.

COUNTING IN SANSKRIT

The Sanskrit numbers from 1 to 30 are as follows (pronunciation guide in brackets where the pronunciation is not obvious from the spelling):

1. Ekam
2. Dve (dwee)
3. Trini (tree-ni)
4. Chatvari
5. Panca (pan-cha)
6. Shat
7. Sapta
8. Ashtau
9. Nava
10. Dasa (dash-a)
11. Ekadasa (ek-a-dash-a)
12. Dvadasa (dwee-dash-a)
13. Trayodasa (tray-o-dash-a)
14. Chaturdasa (cha-toor-dash-a)
15. Pancadasa (pan-cha-dash-a)
16. Sodasa (sho-dash-a)
17. Saptadasa (sap-ta-dash-a)
18. Astodasa (ash-to-dash-a)
19. Ekoonavimsatih (ekoo-na-vim-sha-ti)
20. Vimsatih (vim-sha-ti)
21. Ekavimsatih (e-ka-vim-sha-ti)
22. Dvavimsatih (dwee-vim-sha-ti)
23. Trayivimsatih (tray-i-vim-sha-ti)
24. Caturvimsatih (cha-toor-vim-sha-ti)
25. Pancavimsatih (pan-cha-vim-sha-ti)
26. Satvimsatih (shat-vim-sha-ti)
27. Saptavimsatih (sap-ta-vim-sha-ti)
28. Astavimsatih (ash-ta-vim-sha-ti)
29. Navavimsatih (nav-a-vim-sha-ti)
30. Trimshat

USING THE SANSKRIT COUNT DURING THE PRIMARY SERIES

In the directions I give in this section, the 'state of the asana' is when you are considered to be 'in' the asana. At this point the pose is held for five breaths – this is shown in **bold.** The number given in brackets for each asana – for example, '9 vinyasas' – is the total number of breaths and corresponding movements in the posture, from the entering through to the exiting of the posture. For example, '5 vinyasas – 2nd and 4th are the states of the asana' means that there are five breaths and movements altogether in the getting into and out of the posture, and it is on the second and fourth movements that the posture is held for five breaths.

The vinyasa count might not always seem to make sense at first. Firstly, some movements are just not counted (I'm not sure why this is), so I have just included the breath. For example, for Padangushtasana, after the third vinyasa ('trini – inhale – lift chest'), the hands are placed under the feet on an exhalation that is not counted. Prasarita Padottanasana is another asana in which not all of the movements are counted.

Secondly, for the warrior sequence and the sitting poses the vinyasa count assumes that there is a full vinyasa to standing between the poses. So when a posture ends in down-dog, the jump through to the next posture is on sapta (seven). This would be correct if you had started from Samastitihi (i.e. 'ekam – inhale – reach up'; 'dve – exhale – fold down – Uttanasana'; 'trini – inhale – lift the chest'; 'chatvari – exhale – back and down to Chatturanga Dandasana'; 'panca – inhale – Urdvha Mukha Svanasana [up-dog]'; 'shat – exhale – Adho Mukha Svanasana [down-dog]) – seven is where you take the count up again, inhale, jump through, and sit down for the next pose. Likewise, the numbers at the ends of these postures are not included. So, for example, Purvattanasana is listed as having 15 vinyasas, but the count ends at the thirteenth vinyasa: 'trayodasa – exhale – Adho Mukha Svanasana [down-dog]'. This is because the next vinyasas would always be: 'chaturdasa – inhale – forwards to standing, straight legs, lift the chest'; and 'pancadasha – exhale – fold down – inhale – come up to Samastitihi' (this is one of the movements that is not counted). The count then starts back at 'ekam – inhale – reach up', and so on to vinyasa seven, in which you jump through for the next posture.

Many serious students of Ashtanga have attempted to pin down exactly how the vinyasa count works and everyone has come up with something slightly different. I think we have to accept that there is not one absolutely correct way. The sequence has changed over time and Guruji seems to have taught different things to different people at different times. For me this is part of the beauty of it. Like Christopher Robin's 'Enchanted Place' where you can never be fully sure how many trees there are, the vinyasa count can never be 100 per cent correct – it is different and beautiful for everyone.

SAMASTITIHI

Opening chant

SUN SALUTATIONS

Surya Namaskara A

(9 vinyasas – 6th is the state of the asana)

Ekam – inhale – reach up

Dve – exhale – fold down – Uttanasana

Trini – inhale – lift the chest

Chatvari – exhale – back and down to Chatturanga Dandasana

Panca – inhale – Urdvha Mukha Svanasana

Shat – exhale – Adho Mukha Svanasana (5 breaths)

Sapta – inhale – forwards to standing, straight legs, lift the chest

Ashtau – exhale – fold down – Uttanasana

Nava – inhale – come all the way up, hands together

Exhale – Samastitihi

Repeat 5 times

Surya Namaskara B

(17 vinyasas – 14th is the state of the asana)

Ekam – inhale – bend the knees, reach up – Utkatasana

Dve – exhale – straight legs, fold down – Uttanasana

Trini – inhale – lift the chest

Chatvari – exhale – Chatturanga Dandasana

Panca – inhale – Urdvha Mukha Svanasana

Shat – exhale – Adho Mukha Svanasana

Sapta – inhale – left heel in, right foot forwards – Virabhadrasana I

Ashtau – exhale – Chatturanga Dandasana

Nava – inhale – Urdhva Mukha Svanasana

Dasa – exhale – Adho Mukha Svanasana

Ekadasa – inhale – right heel in, left foot forwards – Virabhadrasana I

Dvadasa – exhale – Chatturanga Dandasana

Trayodasa – inhale – Urdvha Mukha Svanasana

Chaturdasa – exhale – Adho Mukha Svanasana (5 breaths)

Pancadasa – inhale – forwards, straight legs, lift the chest

Sodasa – exhale – fold – Uttanasana

Saptadasa – inhale – bend knees, up to standing – Utkatasana

Exhale – Samastitihi

Repeat 5 times

STANDING POSTURES

Padangushtasana/Padahastasana

(3 vinyasas – 2nd is the state of the asana)

Ekam – inhale – feet hip-width apart, fold forward, take your toes, lift the chest

Dve – exhale – fold down (5 breaths)

Trini – inhale – lift the chest

Exhale – place hands under the feet

Ekam – inhale – lift the chest

Dve – exhale – fold down (5 breaths)

Trini – inhale – lift the chest

Exhale – hands on the hips

Inhale – come up to standing

Exhale – Samastitihi

Utthita Trikonasana and Parivrtta Trikonasana

(5 vinyasas – 2nd and 4th are the states of the asana)

Ekam – inhale – step wide with the right foot, left foot in right foot out, arms to shoulder height

Dve – exhale – right arm down, left arm up (5 breaths)

Trini – inhale – come up, arms at shoulder height, turn the feet

Chatvari – exhale – left hand down, right hand up (5 breaths)

Panca – inhale – come up, turn the feet, square the hips to back of the room

Dve – exhale – left hand down, right hand up (5 breaths)

Trini – inhale – come up, turn the feet, square the hips to the front

Chatvari – exhale – right hand down, left hand up (5 breaths)

Panca – inhale – come up

Exhale – Samastitihi

Utthita Parsvakonasana and Parivrtta Parsvakonasana

(5 vinyasas – 2nd and 4th are the states of the asana)

Parivrtta Parsvakonasana is not in *Yoga Mala*

Ekam – inhale – step wide with right foot, turn feet, arms at shoulder height

Dve – exhale – bend the right knee, right hand down, left arm up and over (5 breaths)

Trini – inhale – come up, turn the feet, arms at shoulder height

Chatvari – exhale – bend the left knee, left hand down, right arm up and over (5 breaths)

Panca – inhale – come up, turn the feet, square the hips to the back

Dve – exhale – bend the right knee, bring the left hand down, right arm up and over (5 breaths)

Trini – inhale – come up, turn the feet, square the hips to the front

Chatvari – exhale – bend the left knee, bring the right hand down, left arm up and over (5 breaths)

Panca – inhale – come up

Exhale – Samastitihi

Prasarita Padottanasana A, B, C and D

(5 vinyasas – 3rd is the state of the asana)

Ekam – inhale – step wide and to the side, hands on hips

Dve – exhale – fold forwards, hands down, head up

Inhale – straight arms, lift the chest

Trini – exhale – fold forwards (5 breaths)

Chatvari – inhale – straight arms, lift the chest

Exhale – hands to hips

Panca – inhale – come up to standing

Exhale

Ekam – inhale – arms to shoulder height

Dve – exhale – hands on hips

Inhale – lift the chest

Trini – exhale – fold forwards (5 breaths)

Chatvari – inhale – come up to standing

Panca – exhale – hands on hips

Ekam – inhale – arms to shoulder height

Dve – exhale – interlock the fingers behind your back

Inhale – lift the chest

Trini – exhale – fold forwards (5 breaths)

Chatvari – inhale – come up to standing

Panca – exhale – hands on hips

Ekam – inhale – lift the chest

Dve – exhale – fold forwards, hook the big toes with the first two fingers

Inhale – lift the chest

Trini – exhale – fold forwards (5 breaths)

Chatvari – inhale – lift the chest

Exhale – hands on hips

Panca – inhale – come back up to standing

Exhale – Samastitihi

Parsvottanasana

(5 vinyasas – 2nd and 4th are the states of the asana)

Ekam – inhale – step feet apart, turn the feet, square the hips to the back, bring your hands behind your back in prayer position

Dve – exhale – fold forwards (5 breaths)

Trini – inhale – come up and turn to face the front

Chatvari – exhale – fold forwards (5 breaths)

Panca – inhale – come up

Exhale – Samastitihi

Utthita Hasta Padangushtasana

(14 vinyasas – 2nd, 4th, 7th, 9th, 11th and 14th are the states of the asana)

Ekam – inhale – right leg up, hook the big toe

Dve – exhale – fold forwards (5 breaths)

Trini – inhale – head up

Chatvari – exhale – leg out to the side (5 breaths)

Panca – inhale – leg back to centre

Shat – exhale – fold forwards

Sapta – inhale – come up, hands on hips (5 breaths)

Exhale – release the leg

Ashtau – inhale – lift the left leg, hook the big toe

Nava – exhale – fold forwards (5 breaths)

Dasa – inhale – head up

Ekadasa – exhale – leg out to the side (5 breaths)

Dvadasa – inhale – leg back to the centre

Trayodasa – exhale – fold forwards

Chaturdasa – inhale – come up, hands on hips (5 breaths)

Exhale – Samastitihi

Ardha Baddha Padmottanasana

(9 vinyasas – 2nd and 7th are the states of the asana)

Ekam – inhale – right leg in half lotus, bind

Dve – exhale – fold forwards (5 breaths)

Trini – inhale – lift the chest

Exhale

Chatvari – inhale – come up

Panca – exhale – release the leg

Shat – inhale – left leg in half lotus, bind

Sapta – exhale – fold forwards (5 breaths)

Ashtau – inhale – lift the chest

Exhale

Nava – inhale – come up to standing

Exhale – Samastitihi

Utkatasana

(13 vinyasas – 7th is the state of the asana)

Ekam – inhale – reach up, legs straight

Dve – exhale – fold down – Uttanasana

Trini – inhale – lift the chest

Chatvari – exhale – Chatturanga Dandasana

Panca – inhale – Urdhva Mukha Svanasana

Shat – exhale – Adho Mukha Svanasana

Sapta – inhale – Utkatasana (5 breaths)

Ashtau – inhale – fold forwards, straight legs, lift the chest

(N.b. this used to be: inhale – up to handstand)

Nava – exhale – Chatturanga Dandasana

Dasa – inhale – Urdhva Mukha Svanasana

Ekadasa – exhale – Adho Mukha Svanasana

Virabhadrasana I and II

(16 vinyasas – 7th, 8th, 9th and 10th are the states of the asana)

Sapta – inhale – left heel in, right foot forward – Virabhadrasana I (5 breaths)

Ashtau – exhale – turn to the left, bend the left knee (5 breaths)

Nava – inhale – arms down to Virabhadrasana II (5 breaths)

Dasa – exhale – turn to the right, bend the right knee (5 breaths)

Ekadasa – inhale – hands down, jump both feet back
Dvadasa – exhale – Chatturanga Dandasana
Trayodasa – inhale – Urdhva Mukha Svanasana
Chaturdasa – exhale – Adho Mukha Svanasana

SITTING POSTURES

Dandasana

This is not listed in *Yoga Mala* as a separate asana – it is a transition posture before other sitting postures.

Sapta – inhale – jump through – Dandasana (5 breaths)

Paschimattanasana

(16 vinyasas – 9th is the state of the asana)

Ashtau – inhale – reach forwards, hook the first two fingers round big toes
Nava – exhale – fold forwards (5 breaths)
Inhale – lift the chest, hold around outside of the feet
Exhale – fold forwards (5 breaths)
Dasa – inhale – straight arms, lift the chest
Exhale – release
Ekadasa – inhale – cross the legs and lift
Dvadasa – exhale – Chatturanga Dandasana
Trayodasa – inhale – Urdhva Mukha Svanasana
Chaturdasa – exhale – Adho Mukha Svanasana

Purvattanasana

(15 vinyasas – 8th is the state of the asana)

Sapta – inhale – jump forwards
Exhale – place the hands 30cm behind the back – fingers face forwards
Ashtau – inhale into the posture (5 breaths)
Nava – exhale – lower
Dasa – inhale – cross the legs and lift

Ekadasa – exhale – Chatturanga Dandasana

Dvadasa – inhale – Urdhva Mukha Svanasana

Trayodasa – exhale – Adho Mukha Svanasana

Ardha Baddha Padma Paschimattanasana

(22 vinyasas – 8th and 15th are the states of the asana)

Sapta – inhale – jump forwards

Exhale – Dandasana

Inhale – take the right foot into Padmasana, bind right arm behind the back

Ashtau – exhale forwards into the posture (5 breaths)

Nava – inhale – straighten the left arm, lift the chest

Exhale – release

Dasa – inhale – cross the legs and lift

Ekadasa – exhale – Chatturanga Dandasana

Dvadasa – inhale – Urdhva Mukha Svanasana

Trayodasa – exhale – Adho Mukha Svanasana

Chaturdasa – inhale – forwards

Exhale – Dandasana

Inhale – take the left foot into Padmasana, bind the left arm behind the back

Pancadasa – exhale – fold forwards (5 breaths)

Sodasa – inhale – straighten the left arm, lift the chest

Exhale – release

Saptadasa – inhale – cross the legs and lift

Astodasa – exhale – Chatturanga Dandasana

Ekoonavimsatih – inhale – Urdhva Mukha Svanasana

Vimsatih – exhale – Adho Mukha Svanasana

Tiriangmukhaikapada Paschimattanasana

(22 vinyasas – 8th and 15th are the states of the asana)

Sapta – inhale – jump forwards

Exhale – Dandasana

Inhale – fold the right foot back

Ashtau – exhale forwards into the posture (5 breaths)

Nava – inhale – straighten the arms, lift the chest

Exhale – release

Dasa – inhale – cross the legs and lift

Ekadasa – exhale – Chatturanga Dandasana

Dvadasa – inhale – Urdhva Mukha Svanasana

Trayodasa – exhale – Adho Mukha Svanasana

Chaturdasa – inhale – forwards

Exhale – Dandasana

Inhale – fold the left foot back

Pancadasa – exhale – fold forwards (5 breaths)

Sodasa – inhale – straighten the arms, lift the chest

Exhale – release

Saptadasa – inhale – cross the legs and lift

Astodasa – exhale – Chatturanga Dandasana

Ekoonavimsatih – inhale – Urdhva Mukha Svanasana

Vimsatih – exhale – Adho Mukha Svanasana

Janu Sirsasana A, B and C

(22 vinyasas – 8th and 15th are the states of the asana)

Sapta – inhale – jump forwards

Exhale – Dandasana

Inhale – take the right knee out to the side

Ashtau – exhale forwards into the posture (5 breaths)

Nava – inhale – straighten the arms, lift the chest

Exhale – release

Dasa – inhale – cross the legs and lift

Ekadasa – exhale – Chatturanga Dandasana

Dvadasa – inhale – Urdhva Mukha Svanasana

Trayodasa – exhale – Adho Mukha Svanasana

Chaturdasa – inhale – forwards

Exhale – Dandasana

Inhale – take the left knee out to the side

Pancadasa – exhale – fold forwards (5 breaths)

Sodasa – inhale – straighten the arms, lift the chest

Exhale – release

Saptadasa – inhale – cross the legs and lift

Astodasa – exhale – Chatturanga Dandasana

Ekoonavimsatih – inhale – Urdhva Mukha Svanasana

Vimsatih – exhale – Adho Mukha Svanasana

Marichyasana A

(22 vinyasas – 8th and 15th are the states of the asana)

Sapta – inhale – jump forwards

Exhale – Dandasana

Inhale – bend the right knee up to the ceiling, bind the right arm around the front of the leg

Ashtau – exhale forwards into the posture (5 breaths)

Nava – inhale – lift the chest

Exhale – release

Dasa – inhale – cross the legs and lift

Ekadasa – exhale – Chatturanga Dandasana

Dvadasa – inhale – Urdhva Mukha Svanasana

Trayodasa – exhale – Adho Mukha Svanasana

Chaturdasa – inhale – forwards

Exhale – Dandasana

Inhale – bend the left knee up to ceiling, bind the left arm around the leg

Pancadasa – exhale – fold forwards (5 breaths)

Sodasa – inhale – lift the chest

Exhale – release

Saptadasa – inhale – cross the legs and lift

Astodasa – exhale – Chatturanga Dandasana

Ekoonavimsatih – inhale – Urdhva Mukha Svanasana

Vimsatih – exhale – Adho Mukha Svanasana

Marichyasana B

(22 vinyasas – 8th and 15th are the states of the asana)

Sapta – inhale – jump forwards

Exhale – Dandasana

Inhale – take the left leg into Padmasana, bend the right knee up to the ceiling, bind the right arm around the front of the leg

Ashtau – exhale – fold forwards into the posture (5 breaths)

Nava – inhale – lift the chest

Exhale – release

Dasa – inhale – cross the legs and lift

Ekadasa – exhale – Chatturanga Dandasana

Dvadasa – inhale – Urdhva Mukha Svanasana

Trayodasa – exhale – Adho Mukha Svanasana

Chaturdasa – inhale – forwards

Exhale – Dandasana

Inhale – take the right leg into Padmasana, bend the left knee up to the ceiling, bind the left arm around the leg

Pancadasa – exhale – fold forwards (5 breaths)

Sodasa – inhale – lift the chest

Exhale – release

Saptadasa – inhale – cross the legs and lift

Astodasa – exhale – Chatturanga Dandasana

Ekoonavimsatih – inhale – Urdhva Mukha Svanasana

Vimsatih – exhale – Adho Mukha Svanasana

Marichyasana C

(18 vinyasas – 7th and 12th are the states of the asana)

Sapta – inhale – forwards, bend the right knee up to the ceiling, twist to the right, bind the left arm around the right leg (5 breaths)

Exhale – release

Ashtau – inhale – lift

Nava – exhale – Chatturanga Dandasana

Dasa – inhale – Urdhva Mukha Svanasana

Ekadasa – exhale – Adho Mukha Svanasana

Dvadasa – inhale – forwards, bend the left knee up to the ceiling, twist to the left, bind the right arm around the left leg (5 breaths)

Exhale – release

Trayodasa – inhale – lift

Chaturdasa – exhale – Chatturanga Dandasana

Pancadasa – inhale – Urdhva Mukha Svanasana

Sodasa – exhale – Adho Mukha Svanasana

Marichyasana D

(18 vinyasas – 7th and 12th are the states of the asana)

Sapta – inhale – jump forwards, take the left foot into Padmasana, bend the right knee up to the ceiling, twist to the right, bind the left arm around the right leg (5 breaths)

Exhale – release

Ashtau – inhale – lift

Nava – exhale – Chatturanga Dandasana

Dasa – inhale – Urdhva Mukha Svanasana

Ekadasa – exhale – Adho Mukha Svanasana

Dvadasa – inhale – forwards, take the right foot into Padmasana, bend the left knee up to ceiling, twist to the left, bind the right arm around the left leg (5 breaths)

Exhale – release

Trayodasa – inhale – lift

Chaturdasa – exhale – Chatturanga Dandasana

Pancadasa – inhale – Urdhva Mukha Svanasana

Sodasa – exhale – Adho Mukha Svanasana

Navasana

(13 vinyasas – 7th is the state of the asana)

Sapta – inhale – jump forwards into the posture (5 breaths)

Ashtau – inhale – lift up

Exhale – down

Sapta – again (5 breaths)

Ashtau – inhale – lift up

Exhale – down

Sapta – again (5 breaths)

Ashtau – inhale – lift up

Exhale – down

Sapta – again (5 breaths)

Ashtau – inhale – lift up

Exhale – down

Sapta – again (5 breaths)

Ashtau – inhale – lift up

Nava – exhale – Chatturanga Dandasana

Dasa – inhale – Urdhva Mukha Svanasana

Ekadasa – exhale – Adho Mukha Svanasana

Bhujapidasana

(15 vinyasas – 7th and 8th are the states of the asana)

Sapta – inhale – jump the legs around the arms, balance on the hands, cross the right foot over the left

Ashtau – exhale – fold forwards, chin towards the floor (5 breaths)

Nava – inhale – come up, straight legs

Dasa – exhale – fold the legs back into Bakasana

Inhale – lift the hips

Ekadasa – exhale – Chatturanga Dandasana

Dvadasa – inhale – Urdhva Mukha Svanasana

Trayodasa – exhale – Adho Mukha Svanasana

Kurmasana and Supta Kurmasana

(16 vinyasas – 7th and 9th are the states of the asana)

Sapta – inhale – jump the legs around the arms, lower down to the floor (5 breaths)

Ashtau – exhale – bind the arms

Nava – inhale – cross the right foot over the left (5 breaths)

OR

Ashtau – exhale – sit up, put the feet behind the head (left then right), fold forwards

Nava – inhale – bind the arms (5 breaths)

Dasa – inhale – lift up to Tittibasana

Ekadasa – exhale – to Backasana

Inhale – lift the hips

Dvadasa – exhale – Chatturanga Dandasana

Trayodasa – inhale – Urdhva Mukha Svanasana

Chaturdasa – exhale – Adho Mukha Svanasana

Garbha Pindasana

(15 vinyasas – 8th and 9th are the states of the asana)

Sapta – inhale – jump forwards

Exhale – Dandasana

Ashtau – inhale – take Padmasana, thread the arms through the legs (5 breaths)

Nava – exhale – roll round in a clockwise circle

Nava – inhale – come up to balance on the hands – Kukkutasana (5 breaths)

Dasa – inhale – release the arms and lift up

Ekadasa – exhale – Chatturanga Dandasana

Dvadasa – inhale – Urdhva Mukha Svanasana

Trayodasa – exhale – Adho Mukha Svanasana

Baddha Konasana

(17 vinyasas – 8th and 10th are the states of the asana)

Sapta – inhale – jump forwards to sitting, put the soles of the feet together, knees out to side

Ashtau – exhale – lengthen forwards (5 breaths)

Nava – inhale – come up, tuck chin in

Dasa – exhale – fold forwards curving the spine (5 breaths)

Ekadasa – inhale – sit up

Exhale – release the legs

Dvadasa – inhale – lift up

Trayodasa – exhale – Chatturanga Dandasana

Chaturdasa – inhale – Urdhva Mukha Svanasana

Pancadasa – exhale – Adho Mukha Svanasana

Upavishta Konasana

(16 vinyasas – 8th and 10th are the states of the asana)

Sapta – inhale – jump through, legs wide, hold the outside edge of the feet, lift chest

Ashtau – exhale – fold forwards (5 breaths)

Nava – inhale – head up

Exhale – release

Dasa – inhale – lift into the balance (5 breaths)

Exhale – release

Ekadasa – inhale – lift up

Dvadasa – exhale – Chatturanga Dandasana

Trayodasa – inhale – Urdhva Mukha Svanasana

Chaturdasa – exhale – Adho Mukha Svanasana

Supta Konasana

(16 vinyasas – 8th is the state of the asana)

Sapta – inhale – jump forwards

Exhale – lie down

Ashtau – inhale – legs over the head, feet wide apart – exhale – hook the first two fingers around each big toe (5 breaths)

Nava – inhale – roll up and catch the balance

Exhale – lower down, head towards the floor

Dasa – inhale – lift the chest

Exhale – release

Ekadasa – inhale – lift up

Dvadasa – exhale – Chatturanga Dandasana

Trayodasa – inhale – Urdhva Mukha Svanasana

Chaturdasa – exhale – Adho Mukha Svanasana

Supta Padangushtasana

(28 vinyasas – 9th, 11th, 17th and 19th are the states of the asana)

Sapta – inhale – jump forwards

Exhale – lie down

Ashtau – inhale – lift right leg up, hook the big toe with the first two fingers of the right hand

Nava – exhale – lift head (5 breaths)

Dasa – inhale – head back down

Ekadasa – exhale – take right leg out to side (5 breaths)

Dvadasa – inhale – lift the leg back up

Trayodasa – exhale – lift the head

Chaturdasa – inhale – lower the head back down

Pancadasa – exhale – lower the arm and the leg

Sodasa – inhale – left leg up, hook the big toe with the first two fingers of the left hand

Saptadasa – exhale – lift head (5 breaths)

Astodasa – inhale – head back down

Ekoonavimsatih – exhale – take the left leg out to the side, look over opposite shoulder (5 breaths)

Vimsatih – inhale – leg back up

Ekavimsatih – exhale – lift head up

Dvavimsatih – inhale – head back down

Trayivimsatih – exhale – lower the arm and the leg

Caturvimsatih – inhale – Chakrasana

Exhale – Chatturanga Dandasana

Pancavimsatih – inhale – Urdhva Mukha Svanasana

Satvimsatih – exhale – Adho Mukha Svanasana

Ubhaya Padangushtasana

(15 vinyasas – 9th is the state of the asana)

Sapta – inhale – jump forwards

Exhale – lie down

Ashtau – inhale – bring the legs over the head, feet together

Exhale – hook the first two fingers around each big toe

Nava – inhale – roll up into the posture (5 breaths)

Exhale – release

Dasa – inhale – lift up

Ekadasa – exhale – Chatturanga Dandasana

Dvadasa – inhale – Urdhva Mukha Svanasana

Trayodasa – exhale – Adho Mukha Svanasana

Urdhva Mukha Paschimattanasana

(16 vinyasas – 10th is the state of the asana)

Sapta – inhale – jump forwards

Exhale – lie down

Ashtau – inhale – bring the legs over the head, feet together

Exhale – hold the outside edges of the feet

Nava – inhale – roll up and catch the balance

Dasa – exhale – draw the legs and the body towards each other (5 breaths)

Inhale – straighten the arms

Exhale – release, cross the legs

Ekadasa – inhale – lift up

Dvadasa – exhale – Chatturanga Dandasana

Trayodasa – inhale – Urdhva Mukha Svanasana

Chaturdasa – exhale – Adho Mukha Svanasana

Setu Bandhasana

(15 vinyasas – 9th is the state of the asana)

Sapta – inhale – jump forwards, place the heels together three hand-lengths away from thebody

Ashtau – exhale – arch the back up, place the top of head on the floor

Nava – inhale – press down with the feet, lift hips up towards the ceiling (5 breaths)

Dasa – exhale – lower the hips down

Inhale – Chakrasana

Ekadasa – exhale – Chatturanga Dandasana

Dvadasa – inhale – Urdhva Mukha Svanasana

Trayodasa – exhale – Adho Mukha Svanasana

FINISHING POSTURES

Urdhva Dhanurasana

This is not listed in *Yoga Mala*.

(15 vinyasas – 9th is the state of the asana)

Sapta – inhale – jump forwards – Dandasana

Ashtau – exhale – lie down – position hands and feet

Nava – inhale – up into the posture (5 breaths)

Exhale – lower down onto the top of the head

Nava – inhale – lift up again (5 breaths)

Exhale – lower down onto the top of the head

Nava – Inhale – lift up again (5 breaths)

Dasa – exhale – lie down

Inhale – Chakrasana

Ekadasa – exhale – Chatturanga Dandasana

Dvadasa – inhale – Urdhva Mukha Svanasana

Trayodasa – exhale – Adho Mukha Svanasana

Paschimattanasana

(16 vinyasas – 9th is the state of the asana)

Sapta – inhale – jump forwards

Exhale – Dandasana

Astau – inhale – reach forwards, take your feet

Nava – exhale – fold down 10 breaths

Dasa – inhale – head up

Exhale release

Ekadasa – inhale – lift up

Dvadasa – exhale – Chatturanga Dandasana

Trayodasa – inhale – Urdhva Mukha Svanasana

Chaturdasa – exhale – Adho Mukha Svanasana

Salamba Sarvangasana

(13/14 vinyasas – 8th and 9th are the states of the asana)

In *Yoga Mala*, Salamba Sarvangasana, Halasana, Karnapidasana, Matsyasana and Uttanapadasana are listed as having 13 vinyasas. Urdhva Padmasana and Pindasana have 14.

Sapta – inhale – jump forwards

Exhale – lie down

Ashtau – inhale – swing the legs up into the pose (10 breaths)

Ashtau – exhale – bring the legs down to Halasana (7 breaths)

Ashtau – exhale – bring the knees down to Karnapidasana (7 breaths)

Inhale – legs back up to Salamba Sarvangasana

Nava – exhale to Urdhva Padmasana (7 breaths)

Nava – exhale to Pindasana (7 breaths)

Nava – exhale – lower legs down to floor – Matsyasana (7 breaths)

Nava – inhale – Uttanapadasana (7 breaths)

Exhale – release

Inhale – Chakrasana

Dasa – exhale – Chatturanga Dandasana

Ekadasa – inhale – Urdhva Mukha Svanasana

Dvadasa – exhale – Adho Mukha Svanasana

Sirsasana

(13 vinyasas – 8th is the state of the asana)

Sapta – inhale – jump forward to a kneeling position

Exhale – place the head on the floor

Ashtau – inhale – come up into the posture (15 breaths)

Exhale – bring the legs down parallel to the floor (10 breaths)

Inhale – legs back up to Sirsasana

Exhale – Balasana (10 breaths)

Nava – exhale – Chatturanga Dandasana

Dasa – inhale – Urdhva Mukha Svanasana

Ekadasa – exhale – Adho Mukha Svanasana

Baddha Padmasana, Yoga Mudra, Padmasana and Uth Pluthi

(14 vinyasas – 9th and 10th are the states of the asana)

Sapta – inhale – jump forwards

Exhale – Dandasana

Ashtau – inhale – take Padmasana

Exhale – bind the arms behind the back

Inhale

Nava – exhale – Yoga Mudra – fold forwards (10 breaths)

Dasa – inhale – come up, place the back of hands on knees, chin towards the chest, look to your nose – Padmasana (20 breaths)

Dasa – inhale – place the hands on the floor either side of the hips, lift up – Uth Pluthi (10 breaths)

Exhale – come down

Inhale – lift up

Dasa – exhale – Chatturanga Dandasana

Ekadasa – inhale – Urdhva Mukha Svanasana

Dvadasa – exhale – Adho Mukha Svanasana

Trayodasa – inhale – jump forwards, lift the chest

Chaturdasa – exhale – fold down

Inhale – come to standing in Samastitihi

Closing Chant

Ekam – inhale – reach up

Dve – exhale – fold down

Trini – inhale – lift the chest

Chatvari – exhale – Chatturanga Dandasana

Panca – inhale – Urdhva Mukha Svanasana

Shat – exhale – Adho Mukha Svanasana

Sapta – inhale – jump forwards to Dandasana

Ashtau – exhale – lie back – **Shavasana**

SUGGESTED READING

I put together this Sanskrit count from a mixture of sources:

Yoga Mala by Sri K. Pattabhi Jois (North Point Press, 1999)

Ashtanga Yoga by Angelo Michele Miele (Lino Miele, 1999)

Ashtanga Yoga by John Scott (Gaia Books, 2000)

Astanga Yoga As It Is by Matthew Sweeney (The Yoga Temple, 2005)

I also used my memory (quite possibly faulty) of many led primaries while in Mysore and at workshops in London.

Any mistakes are my own.

DEEPENING THE PRIMARY SERIES

When leading an Ashtanga class, it can be helpful sometimes to teach in more of a 'workshop' style, and suggest to your students ways to open and strengthen their body to help with their Ashtanga practice.

This chapter is organised around areas of the body that often restrict students in their yoga practice, such as the hips and the shoulders. The majority of the suggestions here are passive stretches, which work on flexibility. There are also several short sequences of poses, which either work on different aspects of the stretch or make the stretch progressively more intense, as well as some strengthening exercises to help avoid over-stretching. For each group of poses, I specify which postures from the Primary Series they can help.

At the end of the chapter, I give ideas for how you can put these stretches and strengthening exercises together for workshop-style classes based on different aspects of the Primary Series.

HOW TO USE THIS CHAPTER

As with anything, your teaching will be far more effective and authentic if it comes from personal experience and practice, so my first suggestion would be for you to try the strengtheners and stretches given here and check that they make sense to you and that you understand them deeply enough to explain them to someone else.

Think about how you might modify the poses for students with injuries, and how you might use props to make the poses safe and accessible for students who have weaknesses or restrictions in their body. Also, think about how you would make the poses safe without props, if you do not have access to them.

Start with one or two ideas and try adding them to a class and see how that goes. Then plan out a workshop-style class, write out what information you want to pass on to your students, what poses you want to do, and how you will build up the structure. Add in a rough time plan. Do the sequence yourself to see how it feels. Keep in mind that when you are teaching a pose, it takes a lot longer than when you do it yourself. Be prepared to add poses in or take them out if your timing is out.

Then go teach! My experience is that students really appreciate the extra knowledge and ideas you can pass on in this way, and that it can make a big difference to a student's practice.

Note: I have given some technical terms and anatomical information about the muscles being stretched or strengthened and about the movements carried out. If anatomy is something you understand and enjoy, then I hope you will find this information useful. If anatomy makes your brain freeze, then please feel free to skip over these sections.

PROPS

The use of props in general is a contentious issue in the Ashtanga world. Some people feel that to stay faithful to the 'Mysore style' props should not be used. Others feel that if a student has pain or a severe restriction that makes safe alignment impossible for them, then use of a prop is helpful and necessary. You have to make up your own mind about this. In a workshop context props can be very helpful to make the poses accessible and safe for everyone. For the passive stretches it is useful to have access to belts, blocks, cushions and bolsters. In a gym this is often not possible, so you have to get creative. You can use extra mats rolled up instead of blocks and bolsters; I have also used students' socks instead of belts, and various equipment found in the gym, such as foot-balls, instead of blocks.

WORKSHOP-STYLE CLASSES

In a workshop-style class, rather than leading the class through the Ashtanga sequence, you choose an aspect of the practice and go into it in depth. This could be a particular type of movement students often find challenging, such as opening the hips or the shoulders, or forward-folding or back-bending. It could also be a particularly difficult pose, such as Marichyasana D or Supta Kurmasana.

In a workshop-style class:

- Start the class with the sun salutations and standing poses to help the students' bodies to become warmed up and their minds to become focused.
- Introduce the class with an explanation of why the pose or movement can be problematic in a yoga practice.

For example, if students find Marichyasana D challenging it could be because:

- o the hips are tight, which makes the lotus pose difficult
- o the muscles down the side of the ribcage are tight, which makes it hard to twist
- o the shoulders are tight, which makes it hard to bind

- Explain to the class the structure of the workshop. For example, if you were working on Marichyasana D you might:

- o start by doing various hip openers to help with Padmasana
- o go on to stretch the muscles that can restrict a twist
- o continue with a series of shoulder openers
- o conclude by looking at ways of modifying the pose that also help individual students work on the aspect of the pose that is a particular challenge for them

- It is also helpful to explain common pitfalls and how to avoid them. In our Marichyasana D example:

- o hurting the knee trying to force Padmasana before the body is ready o hurting the lower back trying to bind before it is possible to twist with correct alignment

- Explain correct techniques for getting into and out of the posture
- It can also be helpful to pass on to students what senior teachers have written about the poses. There are several books about Ashtanga that give useful information: *Yoga Mala* by Sri K. Pattabhi Jois and John Scott's *Ashtanga Yoga* are especially helpful for this. David Swenson's *Ashtanga Yoga: The Practice Manual* is very good for modifications.

I give further examples of workshop-style classes at the end of the chapter.

PASSIVE STRETCHES

Ashtanga is a dynamic form of asana practice that creates a lot of heat in the body, which is good for stretching muscle tissue. However, to stretch also the connective tissue (fascia) that covers the muscles (as well as everything else inside the body) it can be very effective to supplement an Ashtanga practice with a slower, more passive kind of yoga. Connective tissue can become hardened, which can restrict flexibility.

It needs to be stretched carefully because it has little blood supply, which means that if it is injured it can take a long time to heal and it may permanently lose its elasticity and effectiveness.

Here are some guidelines for safe practice of the passive stretches given in this section.

Be cool: These asana should be done when the body is not warmed up. When the body is warm the muscle will stretch, but when it is cold it is easier to access the connective tissue.

Be still: There should be stillness within the posture. Movement engages the muscles, but the aim here is to keep the muscle out of the equation and work on the connective tissue. If there is strong discomfort in the posture, and you feel the need to adjust then do so slowly, keeping movement to a minimum.

Take your time: The passive stretching postures should be held for a minimum of 1 minute and a maximum of 20. They are often held for 5 minutes. Do the strengthening poses for as long as it is comfortable and build up the time progressively.

Go to your edge: As with any asana work, go to your edge (where you feel a comfortable stretch) and no further. Because the postures are held for so long, it is best not to start close to your edge so that the posture can be held for 5 minutes without moving. This is a matter of personal experimentation.

Listen to your body: As with all asana, sensations in your body and your intuition will tell you what is a safe stretch: a sharp pain, especially in the knees or the spine, is the body saying 'no!' and an electrical sensation or fizzing is the body saying 'enough now, stop!' If the sensation continues when you have finished the asana, then you probably did too much, so back off next time. Know the difference between muscles stretching and bone-on-bone contact. There will come a point in any stretch where you reach the limit for your body, a point when you are no longer stretching muscles but just pressing bone on bone. It is important when you have reached your natural limit in a stretch that you accept it and stop. A dull ache in the middle of the muscle is usually OK. Tune in to what is happening in order to work out what is a safe stretch for you.

Work on awareness: When stretching passively, work on awareness, focus and patience. You can do this by using simple meditation techniques, such as holding the awareness on the breath or on the sensations felt in the body.

Don't forget alignment: In passive postures, there is a need for correct alignment but it is much softer than in a dynamic

practice. Allow the muscles to relax so there is the minimum amount of engagement needed to stay in the posture.

Ban the bandhas: In passive stretching don't use bandhas. This is because the idea is to be as relaxed and passive as possible. While some muscle engagement is necessary to hold the shape of the pose and to ensure safe alignment, it should be kept to a minimum to facilitate the idea of letting go, relaxing and allowing the stretch to happen. Also, bandhas create heat in the body and passive stretching is more effective when done cold.

Breathe gently: Use a very gentle, subtle ujjayi breath.

When your students get into a posture, give them the following instructions:

• First check the sensations are not too intense and you haven't gone too far into the posture.

• Then check you have relaxed everything you can – be especially careful to relax your abdomen, your shoulders and your face.

• Use props. It is often useful to support the head or the chest on a cushion so the neck can be relaxed. If there is discomfort or there are old injuries in the hips or the knees, then support the legs. If there is discomfort in the back during back-bending, then support the back. Build up a pile of cushions or foam blocks if necessary. Examples are given in the individual stretches in this chapter.

- Then breathe.

OPENING THE HIPS

I have divided the hip-opening movements into deep lateral rotators, hip flexors and deep hip flexion. I then give some poses that are fun to play with and that also help to open the hips.

Deep lateral rotators

Anatomy: external rotation of the hip

The postures these stretches can help with are:

- Ardha Baddha Padma Paschimattanasana
- Marichyasana A, B, C and D
- Kurmasana
- Garbha Pindasana

Eye of the needle

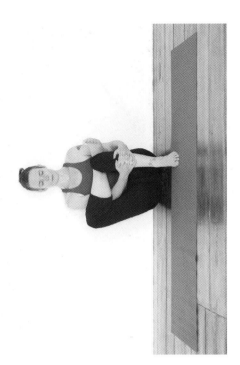

Sit with your back against a wall: this will stop sinking in the lower back. Bend up the left knee. Place the right ankle on the left thigh. The closer you draw the left foot towards you, the more intense the stretch. Make sure the top foot is in a neutral position.

Then fold forwards, using a bolster to support your head if necessary.

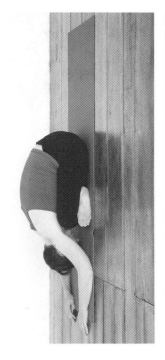

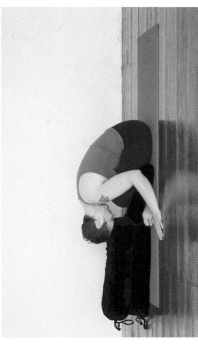

Square pose

Either cross the legs or place one foot over the other knee. If possible place the heels under the knees. Make sure the ankle is in a neutral position.

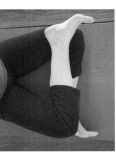

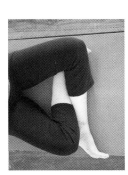

If there is pain in the ankle, knee or hip, support the leg with a block or a bolster.

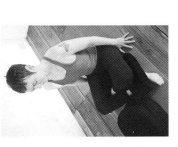

Pigeon

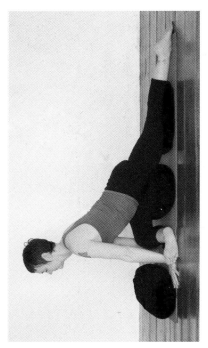

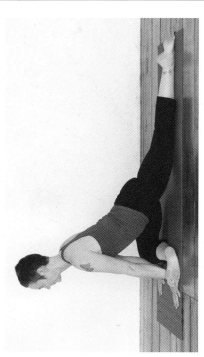

From down-dog step the right foot forwards so the foot is next to the left hand and the knee is just beyond the right wrist. Place the shin on the floor parallel to the hips. So long as there is no pain in the knee, keep the shin in this position and don't let the foot slide down towards the hips. Now lower the hips down towards the floor as far as comfortable. The stretch should be felt in the hip, not in the knee. Engaging the front foot brings more stability into the bent knee.

Many students will require the hips to be propped up on a block or cushions to keep the hips parallel to the floor and the back leg straight out behind.

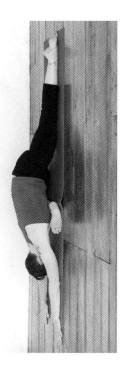

To intensify the stretch, fold forwards.

Hip flexors

Anatomy: hip extension and lengthening the iliopsoas, sartorius, quadriceps, pectinaeus, adductor longus and brevis, gracillis.

The postures this sequence can help with are:

- Tiriangmukhaikapada Paschimattanasana
- Supta Padangushtasana
- Urdhva Dhanurasana

Dragon

To focus on the hip flexors, lunges are very helpful. This sequence of three postures builds up the stretch in the hip flexors very nicely.

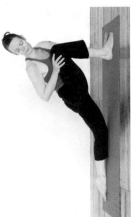

From down-dog step the right foot forwards between the hands. Place the back knee on the floor. Point the back toes

away from you. Relax forwards into the front of the left hip and breathe deeply. Keep the front knee directly above the ankle. If the back knee is uncomfortable, put a cushion underneath.

Add a twist: place the right hand on the right thigh and twist towards the right leg.

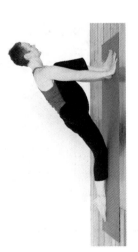

Lift up the back foot and draw the foot towards the hips. This takes the stretch over two joints (the knee and the hip), and so makes it more intense.

Deep hip flexion

The postures these stretches can help with are:

- Marichyasana A, B, C and D
- Supta Kurmasana
- Bhujapidasana

Knee to chest

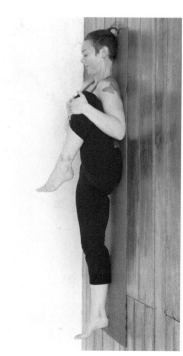

Hug the knee towards the chest, keeping the other leg stretched out along the floor. Take the knee slightly out to the side so the knee aims towards the shoulder. Do the right side first so the ascending colon is stimulated before the descending.

Happy baby

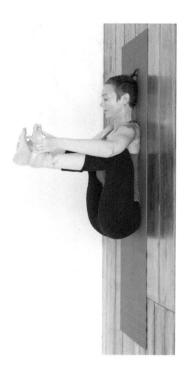

Lie back and point the soles of the feet up towards the ceiling. Take hold of the sides of the feet and gently pull the knees towards the floor on either side of the body. Keep the lower legs vertical and the sacrum down on the floor to stabilise the posture.

Lizard

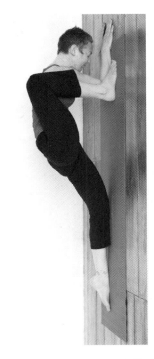

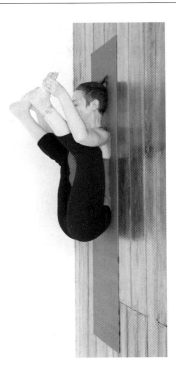

From down-dog step the right foot forwards and point the toes of the back foot away from you. Place a cushion under the back knee if necessary. Make sure the front knee stays directly above the ankle. Lower the chest towards the floor and if possible place your forearms on the floor.

To take the stretch more into the hamstrings, keep the knees where they are and draw the feet down towards the floor either side of the head.

Squat

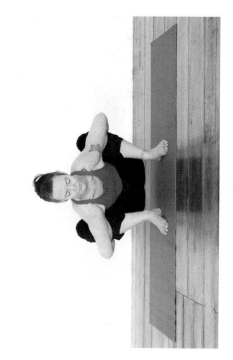

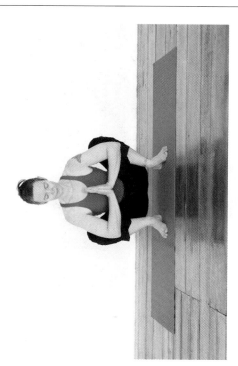

With the feet hip-distance apart and the toes slightly turned out, squat down. Press the elbows back against the knees and lift up through the spine. If the heels are off the ground, you can place a block or a rolled-up mat underneath them. Gently work the heels down towards the floor. Once the heels are down, then take the weight into the balls of the feet.

Add a bind to work on the shoulders at the same time.

Postures to play with

These two postures are not really accessible to most people, but they are fun to try. Offer them to your students in a playful, let's-have-a-go manner.

Titthibasana

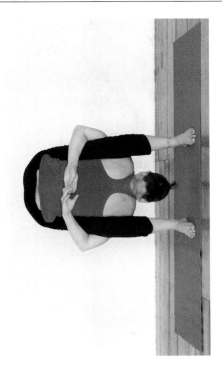

Place the feet about mat-width apart. Fold forwards and take hold of the calf muscles. Draw the shoulders as far as comfortable through the legs. Then fold the arms behind the back and catch your hands. If the hands do not meet then use a belt.

Bird of paradise

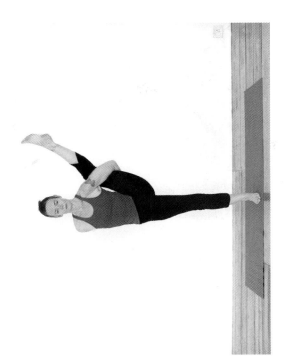

Place the feet about mat-width apart. Fold forwards and take hold of the calf muscles. Draw the shoulders as far as comfortable through the legs. Then bind the arms around one leg. Shift the weight to the other foot and come up to standing on that leg. Straighten the leg that is up in the air.

OPENING THE LEGS

I have divided the leg-opening movements into abductors, adductors, hamstrings and quadriceps.

Abductors

The postures this stretch can help with are:

- Utthita Trikonasana
- Parivrtta Trikonasana
- Utthita Parsvakonasana
- Parivrtta Parsvakonasana
- Parsvottanasana
- Ardha Baddha Padma Paschimattanasana
- Janu Sirsasana
- Marichyasana B and D
- Baddha Konasana

Gomukasana

Fold the right leg over the left leg and bring the foot as far round the side of the hips as comfortable. If possible, fold up the left leg and bring the foot as far round the hips as comfortable. Eventually the feet may be on either side of the hips. Fold forwards.

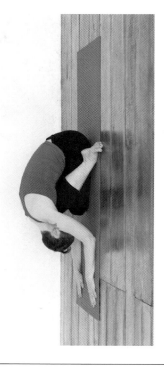

Many students will benefit from sitting on blocks to avoid straining the sensitive lower back area. If the pose is challenging, practising with one leg at a time can be more comfortable.

Adductors

The postures these stretches can help with are:

- Baddha Konasana
- Kurmasana
- Supta Padangushtasana (when the leg is out to the side)

Supta Baddha Konasana

Lie with a bolster under the spine. Make sure the head is supported. Bring the soles of the feet together and knees out to the side. Taking the arms over the head adds a nice shoulder stretch.

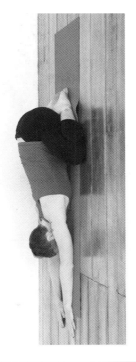

If there is strong sensation in the knees or the hips, prop them up on bolsters.

Frog (Kermitasana)

Place the feet together and knees wide apart and fold forwards.

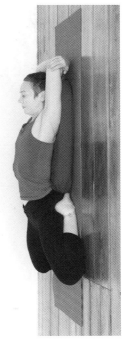

A bolster can be placed under the hips and chest if necessary.

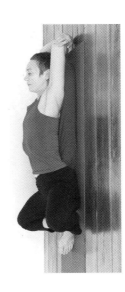

Frog can also be practised lying back.

Hamstrings

The postures this stretch can help with are:

- Paschimattanasana
- Ardha Baddha Padma Paschimattanasana
- Tiriangmukhaikapada Paschimattanasana
- Janu Sirsasana
- Kurmasana
- Upavishta Konasana
- Supta Padangushtasana
- Ubhaya Padangushtasana
- Urdhva Mukha Paschimattanasana

Paschimattanasana

This posture can be practised as a passive stretch and held for at least five minutes. It differs from its more dynamic form (when practised as part of the series) in that the muscles in the legs are not as strongly engaged. Most students need a bolster to support the upper body. Sitting on a block will help students with stiffer hamstrings.

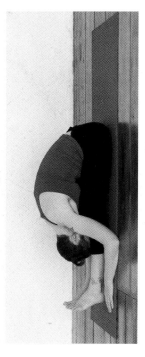

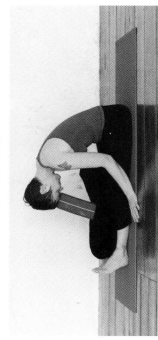

time. The toes should point directly backwards and be next to the body. The knees can come apart, but no wider than the hips. The knees should be allowed to find their natural comfortable position. If the knees are lifting off the floor, then place a bolster under the back. Next, the student should lie back as far as comfortable. Use as many cushions and blocks as needed.

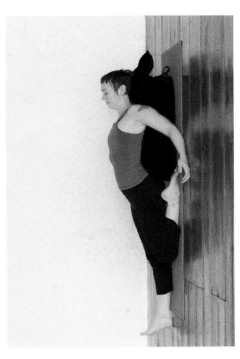

Quadriceps

The postures this stretch can help with are:

- Tiriangmukhaikapada Paschimattanasana
- Urdhva Dhanurasana

Supta Virasana

This is one of the most effective stretches for opening the fronts of the legs.

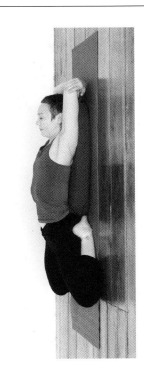

For some people this is a very challenging pose and most people need a block (or blocks) under the hips. If it is too much to fold both legs back together, then fold one leg at a

OPENING THE SHOULDERS

These stretches can help with any postures where there is a bind, including:

- Ardha Baddha Padma Paschimattanasana
- Marichyasana A, B, C and D
- Bhujapidasana
- Supta Kurmasana
- Urdhva Dhanurasana

General sequence

This is a sequence of four shoulder openers that stretch most muscles in the shoulders and generally open them up.

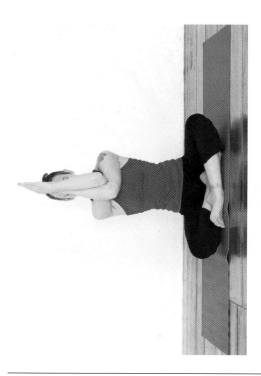

Now cross the arms as high as you can (if possible above the elbows) with the right arm on top, and hug yourself. Point the bottom arm up towards the ceiling. Wrap the top arm round the arm that's pointing up. The thumbs should be next to your face. Press the elbows up and away and draw the shoulder blades back and down.

Take the right arm across the front of the chest. Place the left forearm to the middle of the right forearm. Draw the right arm in towards the chest.

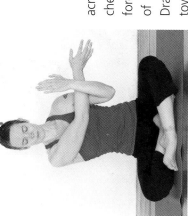

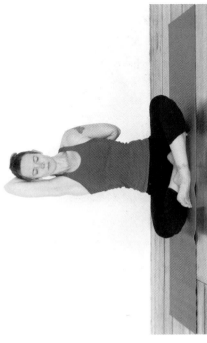

Release the hands and straighten the arms out in front of you, keeping them crossed. Bring the palms of the hands together by rotating the arms inwards. The thumbs should be pointing down and the right hand over the left. Bring the arms up so that the head is between the arms. Gently press the hands together and draw the shoulder blades down.

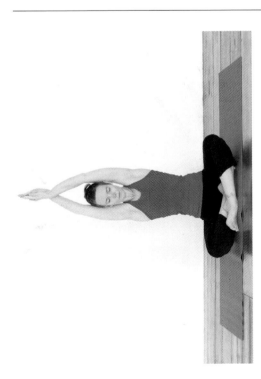

Finally, release the hands and drop the right arm down the back with the middle finger pointing down the spine. Stretch the left arm out to the left side, turn the thumb down and, bending the elbow, bring the back of the hand to the back of the body. Slide the left hand up the spine and clasp the hands behind the back. Relax the shoulders and bring them back towards being level in a neutral position.

If this is not possible, place the left hand on the right upper arm just above the right elbow and use it to ease the right arm down the back.

Dolphin

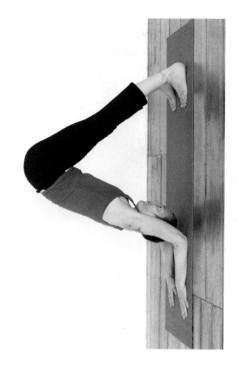

This is essentially down-dog with the forearms down on the floor. Take the chest towards the knees. If it is too intense for the hamstrings, then bend the knees.

Wall hanging

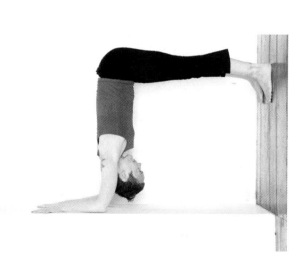

Place your forearms against the wall, keeping them parallel. Fold forwards so your body and legs are at right angles and your body is parallel to the floor. Make sure you don't flare the front of the ribcage down towards the floor. Relax the head through the arms.

Football fan

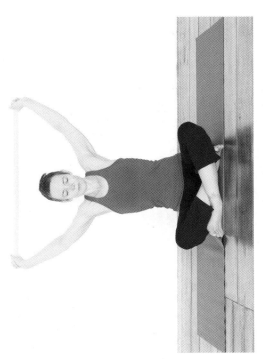

Hold a belt in your hands and stretch the arms backwards. Make sure you keep the front of the ribcage down towards the hips. The closer the hands, the more intense the stretch.

Trapezius stretch

Lie on your back. Place one hand under your body, palm facing down, at the level of the waist. The fingers don't quite touch the spine. Bend up the opposite knee. Roll towards the bent arm. The further over you roll, the more intense the stretch. If necessary, use a cushion under your head.

Rotator-cuff stretch

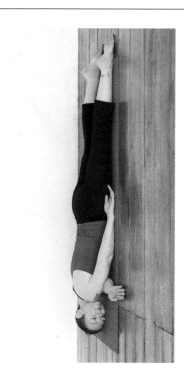

Lie in sphinx (see page 166), then thread the right arm under the body, palm facing up. Make sure you don't go too far and twist. Bring the chest down towards the floor keeping the shoulders parallel to the floor. Place the other arm down by your side, palm facing up.

Pectoral stretch

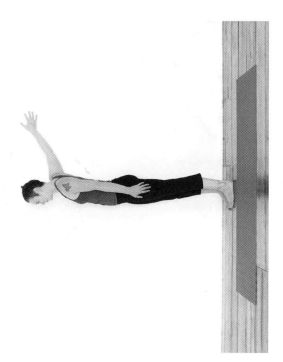

Stand sideways-on to a wall. Place your hand on the wall above your head. Slowly walk your hand down the wall be-hind you until it is parallel to the floor. Keep the chest facing forwards.

OPENING THE WHOLE FRONT OF THE BODY

The postures this stretch can help with are:

- Urdhva Mukha Svanasana

- Urdhva Dhanurasana

Brickwork

Lie with a block under the sacrum. Start with the lowest elevation and spend a few minutes relaxing there. Then take it up to the middle level. Finally, if you feel comfortable, take it to the highest level. Work your way back down in the same way spending a few minutes at each level. Lie flat with knees bent up and the feet flat down on the floor for a few breaths.

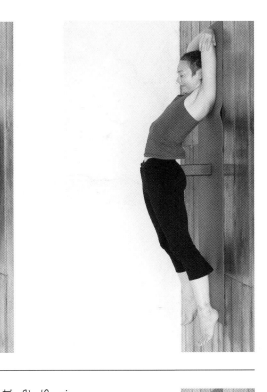

OPENING THE SIDES OF THE BODY

The postures these stretches can help with are:

- Marichyasana C and D
- Bhujapidasana
- Supta Kurmasana
- Urdhva Dhanurasana.

Standing twist

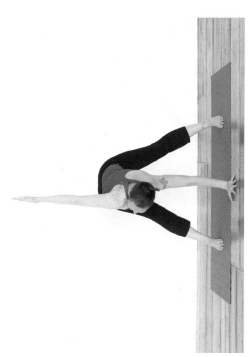

Keep the hips level and twist the thoracic spine.

Twisted pigeon

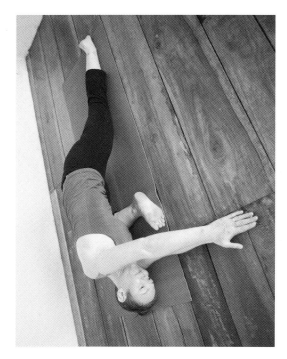

From pigeon posture add a twist to work on the rotation needed in the hips and shoulders for Bhujapidasana and Supta Kurmasana.

Upper-back stretch

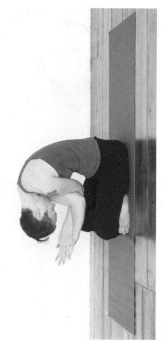

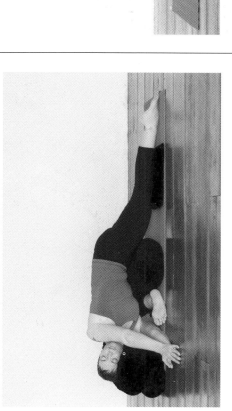

Garudasana arms with a curved forward bend opens the back of the shoulders (trapezius) for Bhujapidasana and Supta Kurmasana.

If necessary, use bolsters to support you so that you can relax and soften into the pose and it is comfortable to hold for 5 minutes.

OPENING THE WRISTS

The postures these stretches can help with are:

- Urdhva Mukha Svanasana
- Bhujapidasana
- Urdhva Dhanurasana

Flexibility in the wrists is important for all postures where the weight is on the hands. If there is pain in the wrists, it can be due to tightness in the muscles in the forearms. If that is the case these stretches will help.

Wrist-bending

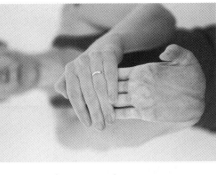

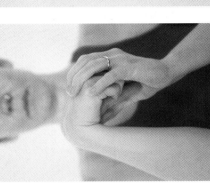

First make a loose fist, then with the other hand, gently draw the hand down towards the inside of the forearm arm. This will stretch the muscles on the outside of the forearm.

Next make a 'stop sign', hold the top of the fingers with the other hand, and press the wrist away from you. This will stretch the muscles on the inside of the forearm.

Then increase the rotation of the hands, (left hand anti-clockwise and right hand clockwise) until the fingers point directly back towards you (or as close as is comfortable). Again, bend the elbows towards the tips of the fingers. This stretch also works on the inside of the forearms, but in a slightly different way.

Fingertips

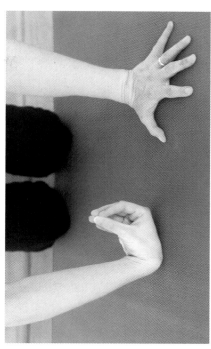

Place the back of the right wrist on the floor, without taking any weight into it. Bring the fingertips together, then release. Repeat several times, then swap to the left hand. This stretches the muscles in the back of the hand and forearm.

Finger pointing

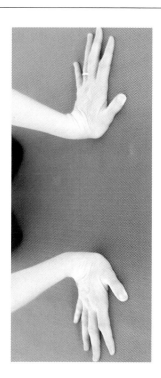

Kneel down comfortably and place the hands flat on the floor, shoulder width apart. Rotate the hands away from each other so that the fingers point straight out to the side (the left hand rotates anti-clockwise and the right hand clockwise). Now bend the elbows towards the tips of the fingers to stretch the inside of the forearm.

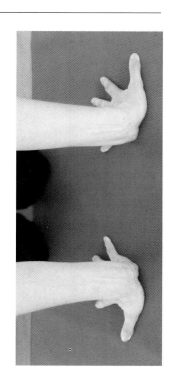

STRENGTHENING EXERCISES

As we increase our flexibility through passive stretching it is important to build up strength, otherwise we can end up over-stretched and weak and therefore prone to injury. Strengthening poses should be practised daily, initially for a few breaths, then built up slowly over time.

STRENGTHENING THE BACK

The postures these poses can help with are:

- Bhujapidasana
- Supta Kurmasana
- Urdhva Dhanurasana

Shalabhasana

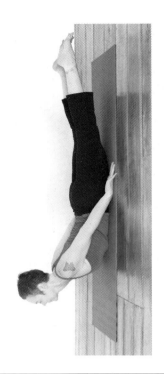

Begin by lifting knees off the ground while the toes press down. With active legs, press the feet together and lift. If there is a weakness or an old injury in the back, lift one foot at a time. Try not to tense the muscles in the hips, use the hamstrings and the muscles in the lower back. Squeeze the inner thighs together.

Dhanurasana

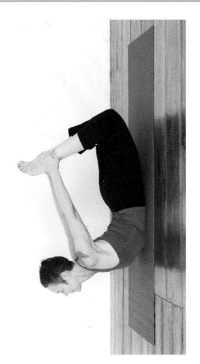

The lift in this posture comes from pressing the ankles into the hands. Again, try not to tense the muscles in the hips. The abdomen stays on the floor, while the hips and ribcage lift up. Keep the feet together.

Superman

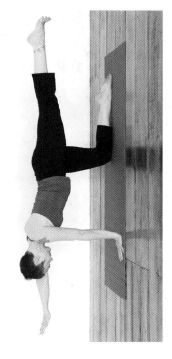

Lift the right leg and the left arm, and then change sides lifting the left leg and the right arm: this diagonal movement can strengthen the core muscles.

Sphinx

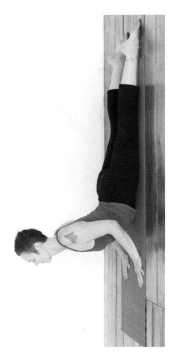

Place the elbows under the shoulders with the forearms parallel. This posture should be active. Without actually moving the arms, make the action of dragging the forearms towards the feet. Draw the shoulder blades down the back to activate the latissimus dorsi. Lift through the chest.

Cobra

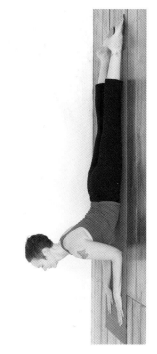

Place the hands underneath the shoulders. Press into the hands to lift the upper body off the floor. Repeat without pressing into the hands, but rather just use the muscles in the back to create lift. Keep the deep hip muscles and gluteus muscles relaxed.

STRENGTHING THE ARMS

The postures these poses can help with are:

- Sun salutations
- Bhujapidasana
- Kurmasana
- Urdhva Dhanurasana

Bakasana

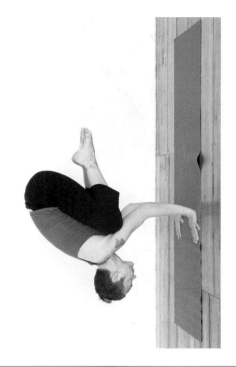

Take care with the wrists in this posture. Ensure the fingers are spread out and keep even, gentle pressure through each finger and each thumb. Place the knees as high up the arms as possible and slowly take the weight forwards. Look forwards. Then, one foot at a time, play with the possibility of lifting up into the balance. Once comfortably in the posture, bring the feet together, and lift the feet up towards the hips. Round the back up towards the ceiling.

STRENGTHENING THE HIP FLEXORS

These poses can help with Urdhva Dhanurasana.

High lunge

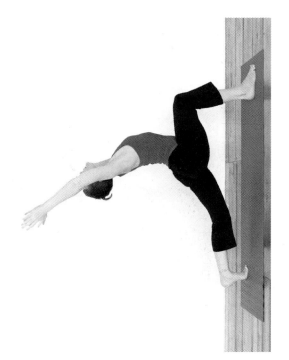

Keep the front knee directly over the ankle. Lift up the back heel and press back into it. Keep the front of the ribcage down. Reach up with the arms, but relax the shoulders down.

High lunge with a back bend

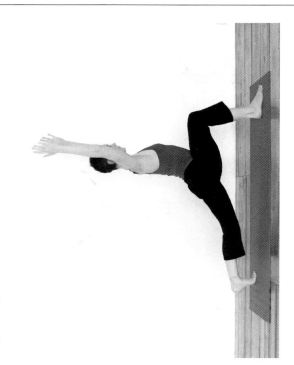

Keep the front of the hips relaxing forwards and bend back from the upper back by lifting the chest up towards the ceiling.

WORKSHOP IDEAS

In the next part of this chapter you will find ideas for five workshops, structured around these key poses: Padmasana, Urdhva Dhanurasana, Marichysasana, Bhujapidasana, and Kurmasana and Supta Kurmasana.

WORKSHOP 3

OPENING THE BODY FOR MARICHYASANA

For all the Marichyasana poses the hips and the shoulders need to be open. The hips need to be open for Padmasana and for deep flexion. The shoulders need to be open for binding. For Marichyasana C and D the side of the body needs to be open for twisting.

Anatomy

Hips: flexion and external rotation and deep flexion

Shoulders: glenohumeral internal rotation.

Side of the body: length in the latissimus dorsi and abdominals

Poses to include

For the leg in Padmasana:

- A selection of the poses given in the workshop 'Opening the hips for Padmasana' – especially important are the deep lateral rotators and, of those, the most important is eye of the needle, which is a very good option to use in class for students who need to modify the posture either

due to stiffness or injury.

For the leg bent up:

- Opening the hips – deep hip flexion: knee to chest, happy baby and lizard

For the shoulders:

- Opening the shoulders: general sequence, trapezius stretch, rotator-cuff stretch and pectoral stretch

For the twist:

- Opening the side of the body: any or all of the poses, especially twisted pigeon, which helps to open the hips as well

Additional information to give

- Many students will need to modify the Marichyasana poses, so explain to your students how to modify safely in a way that will work towards the full posture. If the student's restriction is in the hips, they can do either square pose or eye of the needle. If the restriction is in the shoulders they can do the trapezius stretch.

- Explain the alignment of twisting. The important points are the need to lift through the spine as the twist takes place, and the importance of using the external abdominals to twist and not just push into it with the shoulders.

- Explain that it is important for a student not to try to bind before they can lift up as they twist through the spine, otherwise they will end up twisting with a hunched spine, which can damage the vertebrae and discs.

- It is important not to over twist, shoulders parallel to the side wall is enough. Even if a student can go farther than that, I think stopping at that point is the safest option.

- The neck should also find its natural, comfortable position and not be used to push into the pose – this will just create tension and stress the neck.

Conclusion

The Marichyasana poses, especially Marichyasana D, are a long-term project, and many students will never be able to do the 'full' poses. They can still benefit from the modifications, and opening the hips, opening the shoulders and twisting are all great aspects of the practice to work on. As with all poses, students need to work slowly and gently with awareness to practise safely; this is especially true of Marichyasana D.

WORKSHOP 4

OPENING THE BODY FOR BHUJAPIDASANA

Bhujapidasana is a posture that is challenging for many students. The hips and shoulders need to be open, the torso needs to move in relation to the hips (flexion), and the student needs strength in the arms and the back, and flexibility in the wrists.

Anatomy

Hips: deep flexion, external rotation

Shoulders: all-round flexibility

Torso: flexion

Poses to include

For the hips:

- Opening the hips – deep lateral rotators
- Opening the hips – deep hip flexion

For the shoulders:

- Opening the shoulders: general sequence, trapezius stretch, rotator-cuff stretch
- Opening the hips – postures to play with

For the ability to balance:

- Strengthening the arms: Bakasana

Also include other poses from:

- Opening the side of the body
- Opening the wrists
- Strengthening the back
- Strengthening the arms

Additional information to give

- It is important to be very aware of the foundation of the hands in this posture. Until a student can place the hands flat down, they risk straining or injuring the wrists if they try to do the posture. In a class situation, suggest they work on the two modifications given below and flexibility in the wrists.

working towards. I think it is always useful to share your story with students, let them know when you have struggled with poses and what helped you to work on them.

- To modify this pose safely, I usually suggest either Bakasana (see under Strengthening the arms) or a squat
- One of the keys to this posture is pointing the toes. Once the feet are crossed, point the toes and lift the feet up towards the body
- Then, as the student lowers down, the elbows should slightly bend to control the lowering.
- Students normally progress from going down onto the top of their head, then landing lightly on the chin, then hovering with the chin just above the floor. It takes a while. It's a long-term project for most students.

Conclusion

When teaching challenging poses such as Bhujapidasana, it is important to stress to students that working on a pose is more important that being able to 'do' it. It is the process of breathing, moving the body, becoming stronger and more flexible, developing mental focus and learning about yourself and your patterns that is important, not being able to jump around and twist your body up like a crazy thing!

On the other hand, being strong and flexible and able to do poses such as this feels good and is something worth

WORKSHOP 5

OPENING THE BODY FOR KURMASANA AND SUPTA KURMASANA

Like Bhujapidasana, Kurmasana and Supta Kurmasana are challenging poses. The hips and the shoulders have to be even more open and for the vinyasa the spine and the upper body have to be very strong. Supta Kurmasana, in particular, is often challenging emotionally as well as physically – students often experience feelings of claustrophobia and panic. Explain that this is normal and often often passes in time. If they find it too much they can always practise modifications, but if they can stay with the feelings, observe them and experience them and allow them to unfold, then this can often be a powerful process of release and a way to increase self-awareness.

Anatomy

Hips: for the legs to go behind the head comfortably, the hips need to have deep flexion and external rotation

Shoulders: glenohumeral internal rotation

Torso: flexion

Poses to include

For the shoulders:

- Opening the shoulders: general sequence, trapezius stretch and rotator-cuff stretch

For the hips:

- Opening the hips: all the hip stretches can potentially help with these postures, but especially the ones under 'deep lateral rotators' and 'deep hip flexion'
- Opening the legs: hamstrings

For the movement of the torso:

- Opening the hips: postures to play with
- Opening the side of the body: twisted pigeon

For strength:

- Strengthening the back
- Strengthening the arms

Additional information to give

- When a posture demands fairly extreme movements in the body (such as putting the legs behind the head), it is very important not to rush as this can compromise the alignment for the posture. If a student hunches the back and shifts the hips backwards, this can make the legs go behind the head sooner, but by compromising the alignment, they risk injury to the sacro-illiac joint and to the knees. Insist to students that they take their time and practise with honesty and integrity (see Chapter 6, Teaching the Spiritual Aspects of Yoga on ahimsa and satya). If alignment is compromised then an injury may not happen straight away, but the wear and tear and strain placed on the body is likely to cause injury sooner or later (see Chapter 5, Injuries).

• As with Bhujapidasana, this pose can be very rewarding to work with, both physically (gaining strength and flexibility, learning balance and developing a connection to core strength) and also mentally (coming to terms with being in a challenging situation). Most people have to confront challenges in life in general – if we can learn to work with them in our yoga practice with focus, calmness and balance, then maybe that can help us in the rest of our lives as well.

Conclusion

Stress to students that it is working on a challenging posture like Kurmasana or Supta Kurmasana that can be a powerful transformative process. If someone arrives at one of your classes and is able to do everything straight away, then that may look and feel beautiful, but perhaps that person does not really grow or learn any lessons. It may be a yoga cliché, but there is a lot of truth in the statement that it's the journey not the destination that is important.

SUMMARY

When teaching an Ashtanga class, it is best to keep to the sequence and the flow. If you are teaching in more of a workshop style, then it can be very helpful to use these stretches to help students work out what is restricting them in postures, and to help them work through the restriction. If your students try these postures, they will feel by the intensity which ones are going to be helpful for their body. The more intense the pose, the more they need it.

As with all yoga practices, it is best to do a little bit often rather than a lot sporadically. Students should start gently and build up over time. If the student feels the stretch too strongly or right in a joint, either at the time or after the practice, then they should back off next time. Emphasise that there is no rush and encourage them to enjoy the process.

It is best to practise these stretches either just before an Ashtanga practice or completely separately. It is best not to break up the flow of the practice by adding postures or taking them away. The Ashtanga sequence is a beautiful and complete practice and should remain as it is.

SUGGESTED READING

Yin Yoga: Outline of a Quiet Practice by Paul Grilley (White Cloud Press, 2002)

Insight Yoga by Sarah Powers (Shambhala Publications Inc, 2009)

Yinsights: A Journey into the Philosophy and Practice of Yin Yoga by Sarah Powers and Bernie Clark (Yoga Matters, 2007)

For awareness exercises to do while in the long-held poses: *Prana, Pranayama, Prana Vidya* by Swami Niranjanananda Saraswati (Yoga Publications, 1994)

For information about postures in the Primary Series: *Yoga Mala* by Sri K. Pattabhi Jois (North Point Press, 1999) and *Ashtanga Yoga* by John Scott (YogaWords, 2009)

For ways of modifying poses in the Primary Series: *Ashtanga Yoga: The Practice Manual* by David Swenson (Ashtanga Yoga Productions, 2007).

ADJUSTMENTS

Adjustments are an important aspect of teaching Ashtanga yoga. If you are learning how to adjust, start with small corrections and focus on foundation. Practise on a friend or an old student whom you trust. Ask them if you can try something out and ask them to let you know if it works or not. If you are going to try the adjustments in this book, it is good to have three people: one to adjust, one to be the student and give feedback, and one to read out the instructions.

Although adjustments should be approached with caution, if they are done well they can be a beautiful way to teach. As with all aspects of your teaching, your guiding principle should be care and compassion for your students.

you start adjusting them. This is so you can get a feel for their practice and they can get used to your style as a teacher.

Strength of an adjustment: It can be difficult to judge how strongly to adjust a student. As I explained on page 183, if they are a beginner or have an injury or have not been practising for a while, then just give a gentle correction. Otherwise, move gently and slowly with the breath and feel for resistance. When you feel resistance, stop, observe the body and listen to the breath. Stop and back off if the body is tense or shaking, or if the breath quickens and grows shallower. Sometimes after a few breaths the student will relax more and you can take them deeper into the pose. If you are unsure, ask if it is OK. If you are still unsure, err on the side of caution. Be gentle.

HOW TO ADJUST

FOUNDATION

Before you adjust someone, check his or her foundation. If the foundation is incorrect, the whole posture will be incorrect and your adjusting it will just make things even worse. Also check your own foundation when giving the adjustment.

Feet

Front to back: There should be even balance between the balls of the feet and the heels. If the student is leaning forwards or backwards, this will cause muscles to tense all the way up the body. Try it: stand evenly balanced in the middle, then slowly tip forwards into the toes and notice which muscles tense up.

Side to side: There should also be balance between the inside and outside edges of the feet. The most common pattern is to lean in towards the inside edges of the feet (overpronation). This will cause imbalance in the muscles on the inside and outside lines of the legs and can lead to uneven tension in the knees, a potential cause of knee problems. If someone has knee problems and they do not know why, always check the feet first.

To check: Have the student stand with the feet hip-width apart and ask them to slowly bend their knees. Notice where the knees track in relation to the feet. If the student is evenly balanced, the knees will track directly over the toes, if they are over-pronating, the knees will angle inwards towards each other. If a student is over-pronating in yoga postures, the likelihood is they will do it when they are walking and standing in everyday life. They need to correct it by lifting up the inner edge of the feet so the knees track over the toes. It will take a conscious effort for a while to correct, but it is worth it.

Hands

If the hands are on the floor, they should be flat down, especially if the student is jumping or taking weight (as in Chatturanga Dandasana and Adho Mukha Svanasana). If the finger joints are off the floor, it will cause tension in the wrists, the arm muscles, and the neck. The tip and base of each finger should be in contact with the floor. Place your hands over the student's hands and gently press down. Or place your finger under their hand and ask them to press down on your finger.

Legs

The legs are part of the foundation for the sitting postures.

The feet should be together, toes pointing up to the ceiling (to hold the muscles in the legs in the correct balance).

The heels should be down on the floor (to prevent hyperextension of the knees).

The quadriceps muscle should be gently engaged. This is to protect the knees. To see why, sit with your legs extended and pick up your kneecap – you should be able to easily wiggle it around. Now engage the quadriceps and try to move the kneecap – you'll find it is held very still. The quadriceps turns into a tendon, which goes round the kneecap; engaging the muscle holds the kneecap still and stabilises the joint and so protects it.

The thighs should be gently rotating inwards (medial rotation of femur).

Your foundation

Always establish your foundation before you start an adjustment. Have your feet in the right position and be balanced and controlled. If you are unbalanced or awkward in an adjustment, you will transmit this to the student.

The student's foundation

Part of every good adjustment reiterates the student's foundation. So reiterating the foundation should be the first contact you make and the last you remove. In standing postures this normally means holding the hips to give stability so they can ground into their feet. In sitting postures it normally involves connecting the sit bones to the floor.

ALIGNMENT

Just as with foundation, correct postural alignment – both yours and the student's – is essential when giving adjustments.

Your posture

Make sure during an adjustment that you do not compromise your own posture and safety. Keep your knees bent and your back straight. Be especially careful when you are bending forwards and taking weight – for example, when adjusting Supta Kurmasana and back bends. Stay as close to the student as comfortably possible, it will be easier for you to adjust and it feels more secure for the student.

The student's posture

Before adjusting someone, also check their posture.

Spine: People tend to have one of two patterns – sway backed, where the lumbar arch is exaggerated, or tucked un-

der, where the lumbar arch is flattened. Each causes a slightly different pattern of tension in the hips and back, and they both cause the psoas to tighten and often cause lower-back pain. Help the student to find a neutral position for the hips and lower back. It can help someone to go to the extreme of each; first exaggerating the arch, then completely flattening it, and finding the neutral position in the centre. As with foot foundation, if the hips are out of alignment in a yoga class it is likely to be a habitual pattern in daily life and will require a conscious effort for a short while to break the habit. It is common for a student to lose the flow in their practice while these habits are corrected. This process only takes a short time and after the correction the practice will flow better than ever.

Head: Check the position of the head. The head is very heavy compared to the rest of the body. It can weigh up to 5.5kg (12lb). The muscles in the neck will be in balance when the head is in a central neutral position. If the head is tilted or the chin thrust forward, this will set up tension and probably cause neck and shoulder pain.

BREATH

Before adjusting a student, make sure they are breathing deeply. If their breath is short or shallow, tell them to breathe slowly and deeply before you adjust them.

Adjust with the breath: For forward bends and twists, back off and give a little space on the inhalation and go deeper on the exhalation. For back bends it is the opposite: give space on the exhalation and adjust on the inhalation.

Breathe in time: Breathe in time with the student so you are exhaling as they exhale. This helps you to tune in and become more sensitive and aware.

TOUCH

Whole hand: Use your whole hand when adjusting – spread your fingers wide and make full contact. Adjusting with your fingertips can feel either too strong or too intimate.

Gentle but firm: A soft feathery touch feels horrible, and so does a rough adjustment. Aim for the middle ground, gentle but firm.

Relax: Make sure you are relaxed when adjusting students. If you are tense that will be communicated to the student through your hands. You also need to make sure the student is relaxed; a tense muscle will not stretch and is more likely to break.

Flow: After a while, adjusting becomes like another yoga practice: you flow with your breath and posture combined with the student's breath and posture. You also flow with the needs of the class.

Body weight: As much as possible, use your body weight rather than your strength.

Sensitive: There are certain areas of the body you should not touch. That is obvious. But there are areas of the body that are sensitive – for example, close to the chest and the groin. You can touch someone here, but make sure your touch is firm and confident: if you fumble or touch too gently it is likely to make the student feel uncomfortable.

ADAPTABILITY

Everybody is different and so every adjustment will be different. Once you are comfortable with the basics, be ready to experiment and play around with adjustments to make them right for each student. For example, if you are much taller or shorter than the student you are adjusting, you will probably have to experiment and adapt. If you are the taller one, try kneeling down; if you are the smaller one, you will need to find a way to use your body weight and get in closer.

A POSTURE-BY-POSTURE GUIDE TO ADJUSTMENT

In the final part of this chapter you will find detailed instructions for those poses in the Primary Series where adjustments may be particularly helpful.

SUN SALUTATIONS

Surya Namaskara

As the student reaches up, gently press their shoulders down to remind them to relax the shoulders.

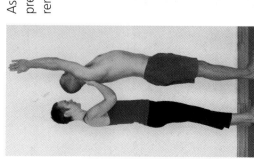

Use your toes to ground the heels and use your hands either to stop the rib cage from flaring upwards or to relax the shoulders.

As the student folds forward, one hand stabilises by pressing down on the sacrum and the other gently presses down the back to encourage the forward bend.

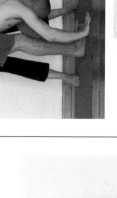

Then step over the student's hips in Chatturanga and hold the shoulders to make sure they do not go down too low.

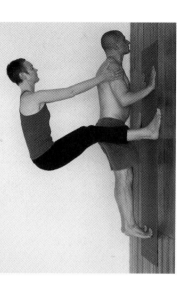

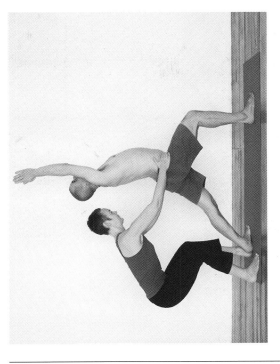

Hold the tops of the arms and rotate them back (lateral rotation of the humerus).

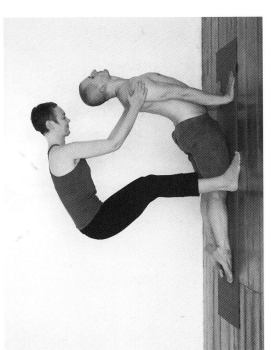

Place your foot behind their foot to stabilise, and use your hands to encourage their hips to square to the front.

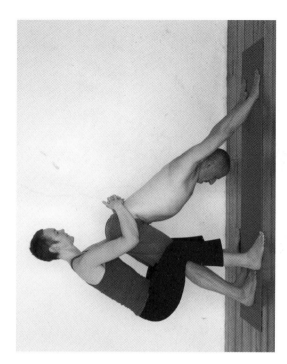

Another way of doing this adjustment is to grip the hips with the insides of the elbows and sink the weight back.

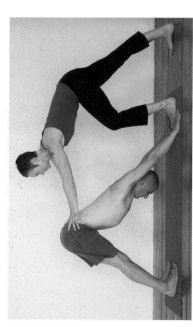

Place your hands over the student's sacrum and press back and up. Sink in with your body weight.

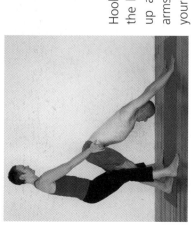

Hook your hands over the hip bones and draw up and back. Keep the arms straight and use your body weight.

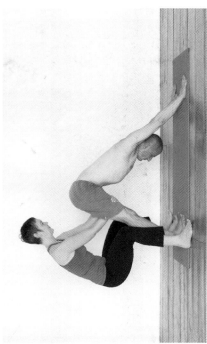

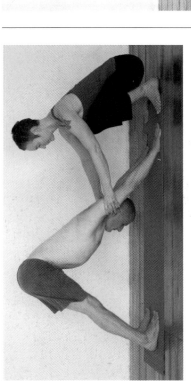

Rotate the upper arms out (lateral rotation).

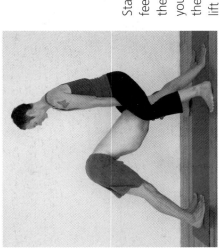

Stand with your feet either side of the shoulders, hook your hands under the shoulders and lift directly up.

For this adjustment, stand either side of the student's feet, put your hands together and thread them between their thighs, then cross the hands and hook them over their mid-thigh and sink your weight back.

STANDING POSTURES

Padangushtasana

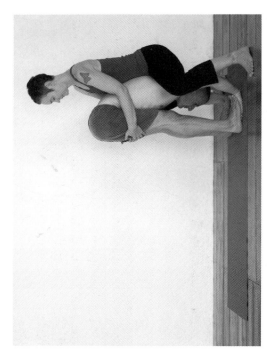

To set the foundation: Place your hand on the student's back (this will be different for each person) and encourage movement down. If you want to add some power to the adjustment, place the inside of your knee over your hand and use your leg to push in and down.

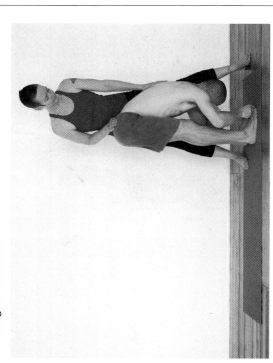

Placement: Stand with your feet either side of the student's shoulders, hold the tops of their legs (or the sides of their hips) and place your abdomen on their back.

To adjust: With your hands encourage medial rotation of the thighs and with your abdomen press gently down and in.

Note: You can feel the breath through your abdomen.

As you finish: Place your hand on their sacrum and press down to steady them as you step away.

Utthita Trikonasana

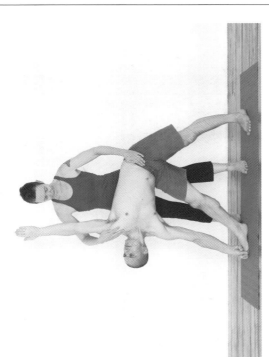

This adjustment works well if the student's alignment is good.

To set the foundation: Place your left hip against the top of their right leg and place your left hand against their left hip so you can hold them securely between your hip and hand. Now place your right hand over their left shoulder.

To adjust: With equal and opposite pressure, draw your hands back towards you and press forwards with your hip.

Also think about creating length by drawing your hands away from each other.

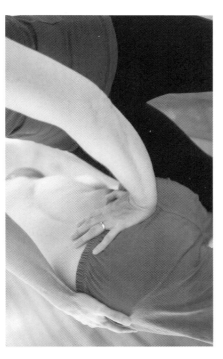

Caution: If the student has sacro-iliac issues, be very cautious about drawing back with your left hand.

This adjustment is for people who anteriorly arch the lumbar spine (stick their tailbone out behind them).

To set the foundation: Place your right hip against the top of their right leg and place your right hand on their left hip.

To adjust: Now place your left hand against their sacrum. The action of this adjustment is to lengthen the tailbone away from the head, so the right hand draws up and back towards you and the left hand presses down towards the floor.

Parivrtta Trikonasana

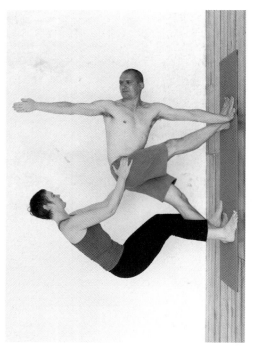

The priority when adjusting this posture is to get the hips level.

To set the foundation: Place your foot on the floor behind their foot.

To adjust: Hook your hands round their hips and draw their right hip back and the left hip forwards so the hips are level.

You can also hold the student's hips and ask them to pull away from you – they can then use the resistance to lengthen and rotate deeper into the posture. Give equal and opposite pressure.

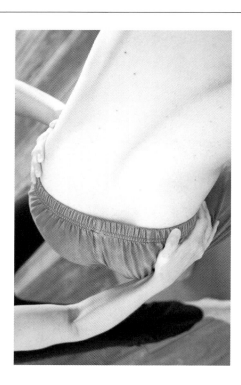

This adjustment is for people whose spine curves up towards the ceiling.

Stand at their feet. Place your right hand so you hook their right hip and your left hand on their left hip – draw your right hand towards you and push the left hand up and back.

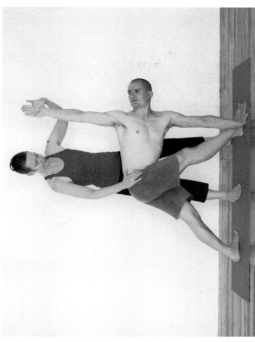

Use this adjustment if the hips are already square.

To set the foundation: Place your right hip against their left hip and your right hand against their right hip.

To adjust: Place your left hand on their left shoulder and your left leg against their ribcage. Now draw your hands away from each other to lengthen the right side of their body.

Also use your left hand to draw the shoulder back.

Use your left leg against the ribcage to encourage the rotation of the ribcage up towards the ceiling.

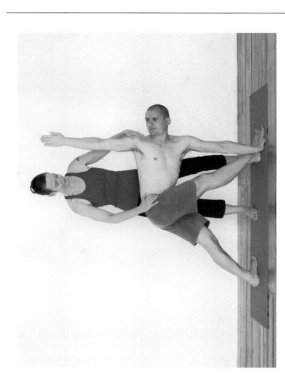

This adjustment uses resistance work to encourage the student to work in the posture themselves.

To set the foundation: Place your right hip against their left hip and your right hand against their right hip.

To adjust: Now place your left hand against their right hand and ask them to press into your hand. Give the student equal and opposite pressure so they can use this resistance to lengthen through the spine and rotate the ribcage up to the ceiling.

Utthita Parsvakonasana

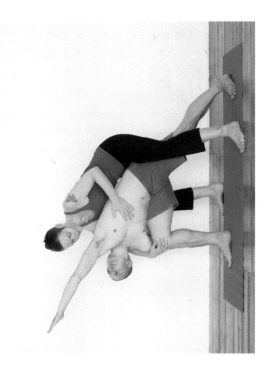

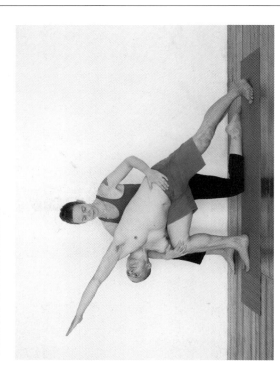

To set the foundation: Depending on your height in relation to the student, it may be best to stand or kneel. Place your left hip against the top of their right leg and place your left hand on their left hip and your right hand on the inside of their right knee.

To adjust: Use your left hip to push the top of the thigh forwards in line with their heel – your hands draw back and away from each other.

You can do this adjustment only on someone of a similar size to you or smaller than you.

To adjust: Stand over the student's back leg and use your left leg to draw the left hip up and back. Use your right leg to press the right hip forwards. Use your right hand to draw the knee back and your left hand to rotate the ribcage up towards the ceiling.

Parivrtta Parsvakonasana

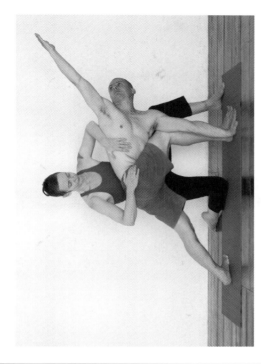

To set the foundation: This is often done by fixing their back foot with your foot. However, if the foot is fixed and the hips are manipulated, then the knee is vulnerable. So to avoid putting pressure on the knee, set the foundation by holding their thigh between your legs.

To adjust: Hook your right hand round the student's right hip and your left hand on the left side of their lower back. The right hand pulls back towards you and the left hand pushes away from you.

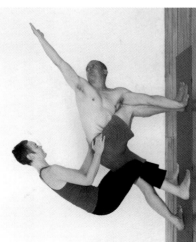

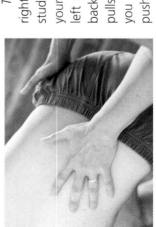

To set the foundation: Place your right hip against the student's left hip and hook your right hand round their right hip.

To adjust: Place your left forearm on the side of their ribcage and your right hand on their hip. The right hand pulls back and the left hand encourages the ribcage to rotate up towards the ceiling.

Prasarita Padottanasana C

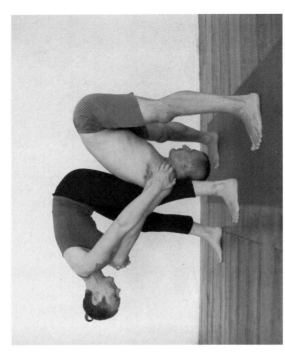

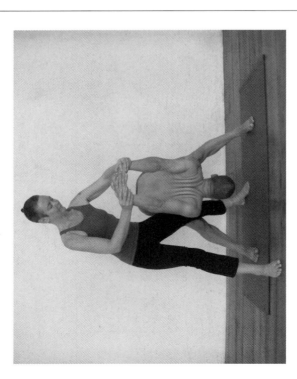

To set the foundation: It is very easy to knock a student off balance in this posture, so as you start the adjustment place your hand on their sacrum and press down. If their hands are quite far from the ground, then step your leg in front of one of their legs. Make sure it is not directly on their knee.

To adjust: Holding their hands, gently press down.

To set the foundation: If the student's arms are fairly close to the floor, then step through their arms so your leg is just in front of their spine. Make sure your other leg steps forwards so you can keep your balance if the student rests their weight on you.

To create more space: Draw their shoulders against the back of your calf.

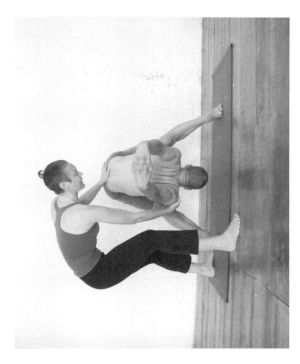

As you step away, to help the student keep their balance, put one hand on their sacrum and the other on their shoulder and help them back up.

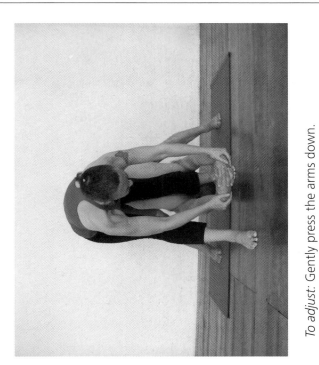

To adjust: Gently press the arms down.

Parsvottanasana

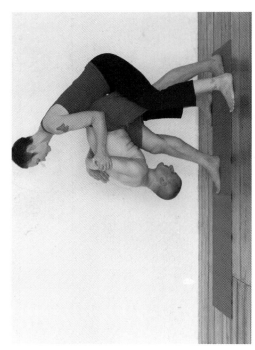

To set the foundation: Stand with your feet either side of the student's hips, place your abdomen on their sacrum and press down.

Note: The only body contact you make is your abdomen to their sacrum.

To adjust: Place your hands over their shoulders and the inside of your arms on the outside of their upper arms. First, draw the shoulders away from the ears, then press the arms in towards each other and lift the elbows up towards the ceiling.

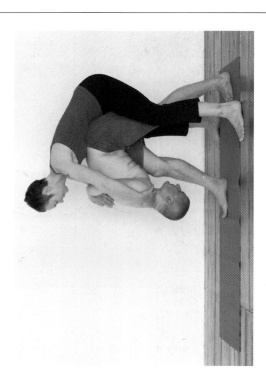

Try this variation if you cannot reach around the shoulders.

To set the foundation: Place your elbows on the side of the student's hips to stabilise and your hands on their elbows.

To adjust: The action is the same as for the standard adjustment – press the elbows in towards each other and lift them up towards the ceiling.

Utthita Hasta Padangushtasana

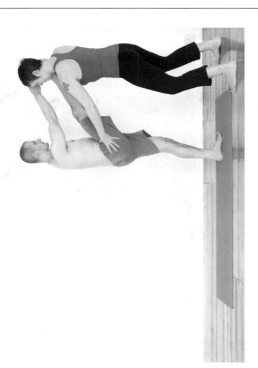

To set the foundation: Stand near to the student's foot – the closer you hold the foot to your body the easier it is for you. Hold the foot with your right hand, and hook the top of the thigh (inguinal crease) with your left hand.

To adjust: With your left hand, encourage the hip back and down, aiming for the hips to be level. With the right hand, gently encourage the foot up.

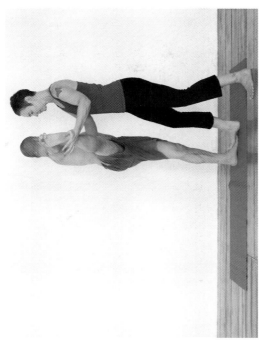

To maintain the student's balance: Move your feet as little as possible and let them take their own leg out to the side.

As the leg goes out to the side, lean back and swap hands so the left hand is now holding the foot, then take one step forwards to place your foot over their foot.

To adjust: Put your right hand to the top of their leg and encourage outward rotation (lateral rotation); the left hand encourages the foot up.

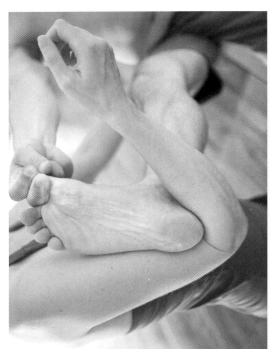

If their leg is heavy, you can hold it in the crook of your elbow – it is much easier for you this way.

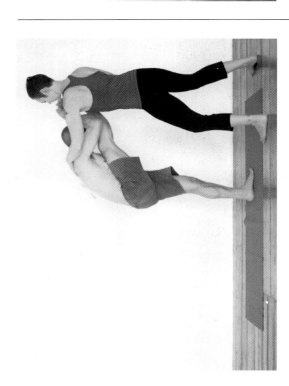

For the final part of this adjustment: Lean back and swap from the left hand to the right as the leg comes back to the front, then place your left hand on their back to encourage the forward bend.

Utkatasana

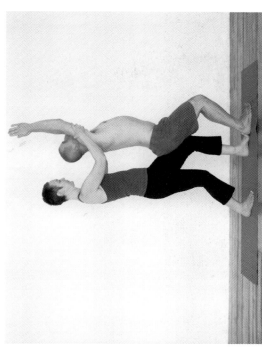

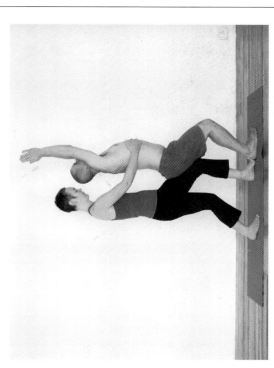

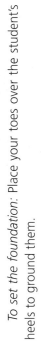

To set the foundation: Place your toes over the student's heels to ground them.

Lower their hips so the student can sit on your thigh.

To adjust: First make sure the hips are in a neutral position, then either draw the front of the ribcage down towards the hips …

… or rotate the arms out (lateral rotation). Another option (not shown) is to soften the shoulders down.

Virabhadrasana I

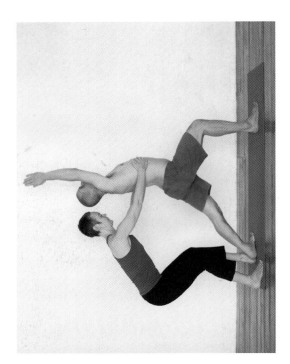

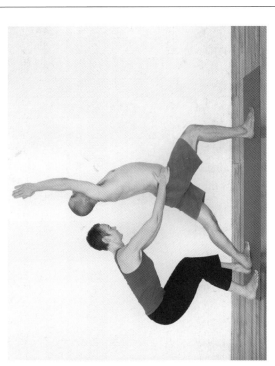

To set the foundation: Place your foot on the floor behind the student's foot.

To adjust: Square their hips by drawing the right hip back and encouraging the left hip forwards ...

... or, if the front of the ribcage is flaring up, draw the ribs down towards the hips.

Virabhadrasana II

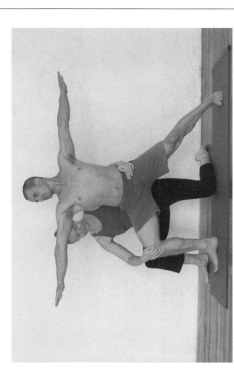

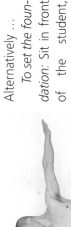

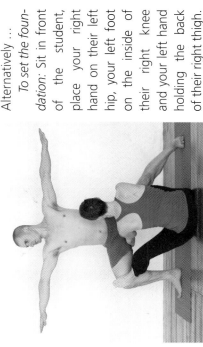

Alternatively …
To set the foundation: Sit in front of the student, place your right hand on their left hip, your left foot on the inside of their right knee and your left hand holding the back of their right thigh.

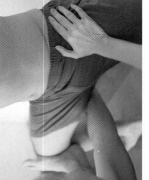

To adjust: Your foot and your right hand push away from you and your left hand pulls towards you.

You can adjust this posture in the same way as Utthita Parsvakonasana because the legs are the same.

To set the foundation: Depending on your height in relation to the student, it may be best to stand or kneel. Place your left hip against the top of their right leg and place your left hand on their left hip and your right hand on the inside of their right knee.

To adjust: Use your left hip to push the top of the thigh forwards in line with their heel. Your hands draw back and away from each other and your hip gives equal and opposite pressure forwards.

SITTING POSTURES

Dandasana

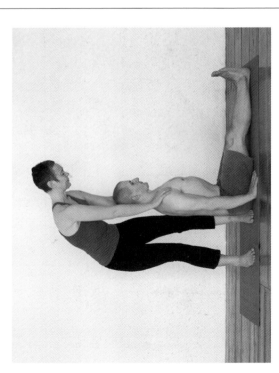

Use the side of your leg to guide the spine upright.
Use your hands to encourage the shoulders to relax down.

Paschimattanasana

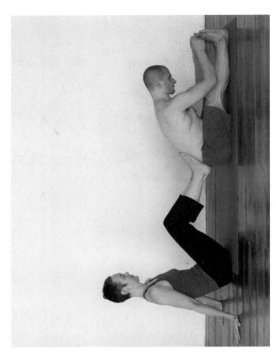

There are several different ways of adjusting Paschimattan-asana depending on the student's level of flexibility. Try this if the student is fairly upright.

To set the foundation: Sit behind them and use your feet on either side of the lower spine.

To adjust: Press forwards and up.

Note: Make full contact with your feet.

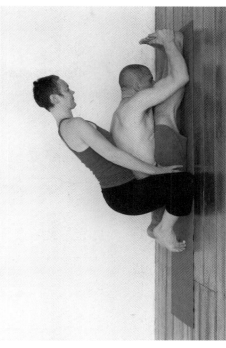

This adjustment works well for students with a medium level of flexibility.

To set the foundation: Use your knees to ground the sides of their hips.

To adjust: Place your hands in the back (below the curve) and encourage movement up and forwards.

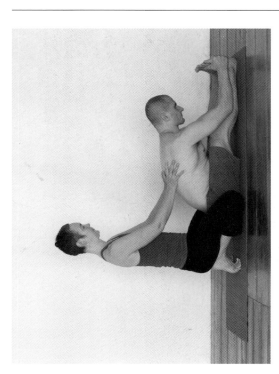

This variation is for students who are very flat down.

To set the foundation: Place your knees on the floor either side of their hips.

To adjust: Place your abdomen on their lumbar area and gently press down – not forwards. Use your hands to encourage the shoulders to relax or bring the feet into the right position.

Note: If a student is very flexible and you continue to push them forwards, there is a danger you can over-stretch the ligaments in the lower back and hips. This can destabilise the sacro-iliac joint. If this is the case make sure you press down not forwards.

Purvattanasana

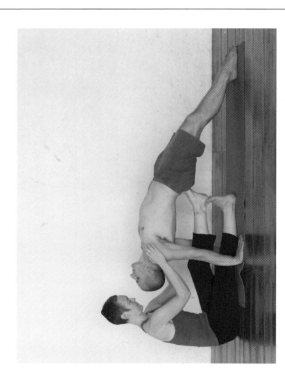

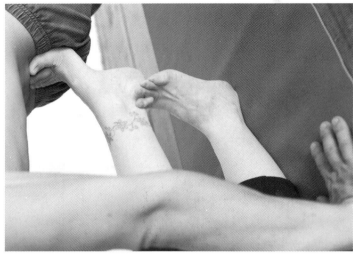

To set the foundation: Sit down behind the student before they go up and place the ball of your foot on their sacrum.

To adjust: As they lift up into the posture, press their sacrum up and away with the ball of your foot.

Press directly down on their shoulders – this will ground them into their hands.

Use one foot under the other for support …

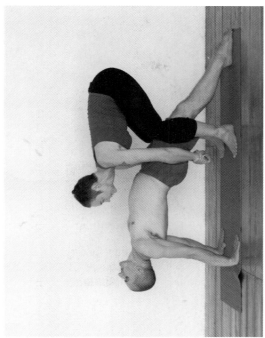

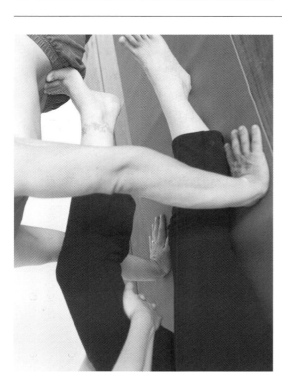

... or, if two feet will not fit, use your hands under your thigh.

To set the foundation (variation): Stand with your legs either side of the student's mid-thigh. Hold one wrist with the other hand and place your hands around the widest part of their hips.

To adjust: Lift their hips up and towards you.

Use your legs to support their weight by squeezing their legs between yours.

Note: Make sure your legs do most of the work to protect your back and shoulders.

Ardha Baddha Padma Paschimattanasana

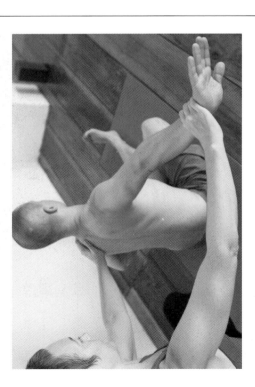

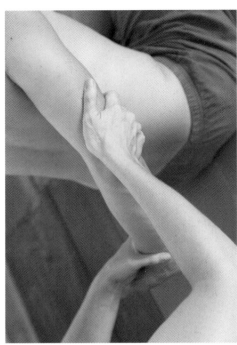

If the student has problems binding but they are fairly close: Put your hand on the opposite shoulder for stability. Then take hold of the student's wrist and ask them to relax their arm. As they inhale, pull outwards as if you are trying to make their arm longer – keep this tension then draw the arm round in a circle.

Swap your hands over, so one hand can guide their wrist and the other can ease their elbow round.

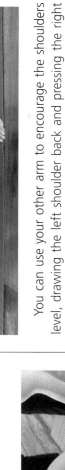

You can use your other arm to encourage the shoulders level, drawing the left shoulder back and pressing the right shoulder gently down.

Note: The focus should be on squaring the shoulders not taking them deeper into the posture.

Keep the pressure on the elbow and use your other hand to place their hand on their foot.

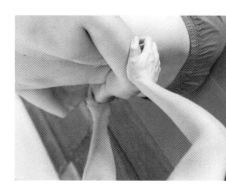

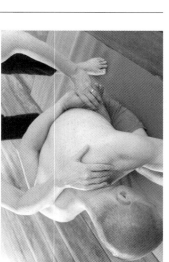

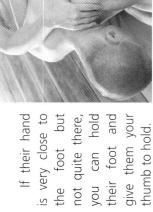

If their hand is very close to the foot but not quite there, you can hold their foot and give them your thumb to hold.

Tiriangmukhaikapada Paschimattanasana

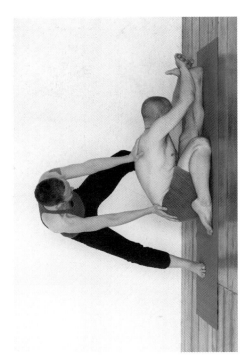

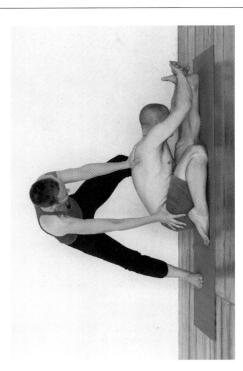

To keep the student upright: Place your left foot on the floor level with their left mid-thigh. Now use the inside of your leg against the side of their ribcage to keep them upright.

To ground the right hip: Place your right hand on the right hip, hooking your thumb where the leg meets the body (inguinal crease), then press directly down.

To take the student deeper into the posture: Place your left hand on the right side of their back and use your left hand and left leg to take them forwards and down.

If they are already fairly far down into the posture, place your left hand on the top of the right hip as shown above.

Janu Sirsasana A and B

Do not do this if the knee is high off the floor.

Do not press down at all – just gently back.

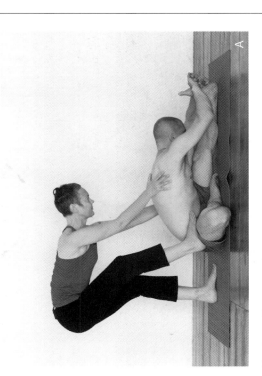

A

For Janu Sirsasana A:

To give grounding: Place your right foot at the top of the student's right leg and use your foot to rotate the thigh back towards you (lateral rotation of the femur).

To correct the student's alignment: Use your right hand on their upper back and your left hand under their lower ribcage to rotate the ribcage towards the straight leg.

To adjust: Ease them gently down into the posture.

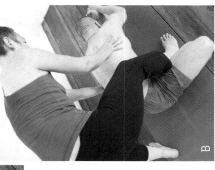

B

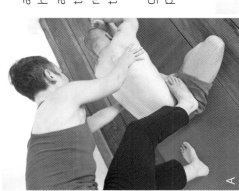

A

For Janu Sirsasana B or if the knee is off the floor for A: Do not place your foot on their leg – just place it in front of the leg to keep it in the correct place.

Then focus on the rotation of the ribcage.

N.B.: Do not adjust Janu Sirsasana C.

Marichyasana A

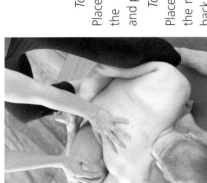

To set the foundation: Place your right hand on the student's right knee and press directly down.

To take them deeper: Place your left hand on the right side of the upper back. Now use your left leg and right hand to take them forwards and down.

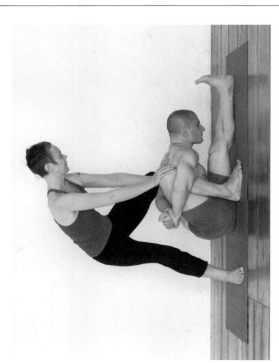

To keep the student upright: Place your left foot level with their mid-thigh and use the inside of your leg against the middle of their left upper arm.

Marichyasana C

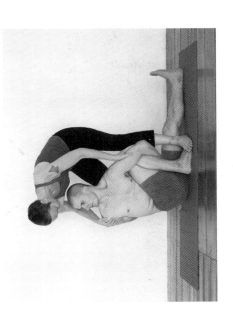

Try this version if the student is already deeply into the posture.

To keep them upright: Place your left leg against the middle of their left arm.

To set the foundation: Place your right hand on their right hip and press back and down.

To take them deeper: Use your left hand (on the right side of their back) and your left leg to take them forwards and down.

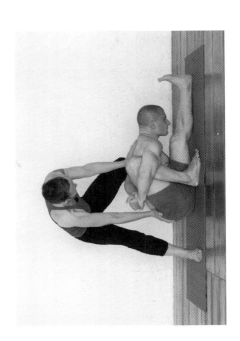

To set the foundation: Place your left foot over the student's right foot (your heel should fit on the floor between their leg and foot). Use the inside of your right leg against the left side of their back to give support and encourage an upward lift.

To keep the bind in place: Place your left hand on their left upper arm and roll forwards and down.

To encourage the twist: Place your right hand to their right shoulder; draw up and back. Encourage the lift on their inhale and the twist on the exhale.

To help someone bind: See Marichyasana D.

Marichyasana D

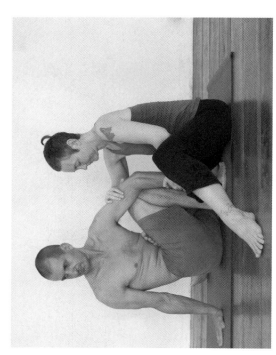

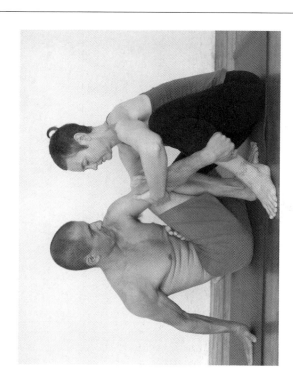

To set the foundation: Sit in front of the student and slightly to their right. Place your right leg over the leg in Padmasana. Do not push the leg down, just hold it in place.

Place your right hand on their right knee to stabilise.

To bind: Take hold of their upper left arm with your left hand. Now pull the arm down so you are bringing the side of their ribcage towards the top of their right thigh.

To keep the arm in place: Use your right hand to rotate the top of their left arm forwards and down.

Use your left hand to guide their arm around their leg.

To set the foundation: Sit behind them and put your left leg over the leg in Padmasana to hold it in place. Do not push down.

Place the left hand just under the curve of their left upper back.

Place your right hand on their right shoulder and your forearm along their upper arm.

To adjust: Your right hand draws the shoulder back towards you and your left hand encourages a lift upwards.

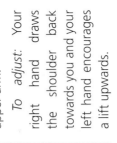

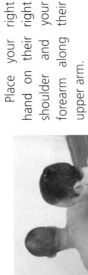

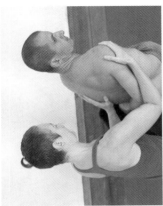

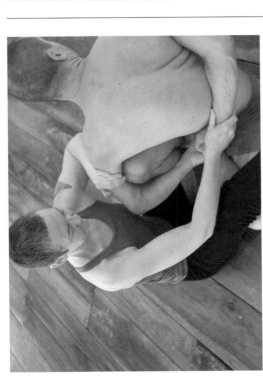

Now swap hands so your left hand holds the upper arm in place.

Use your right hand to draw their other arm round their body and connect the fingers.

Do the following to adjust a student already comfortably in the posture.

Bhujapidasana

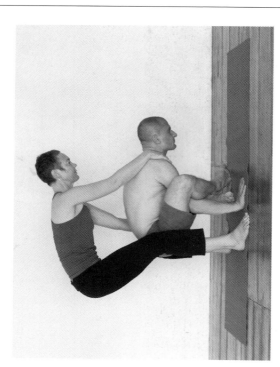

Use this if the student is in the balance but cannot fold forwards.

To set the foundation: Stand behind them so you can support their hips with your legs.

Place your right hand on their right shoulder.

Place your left hand under their left thigh.

Help them fold forwards.

Kurmasana

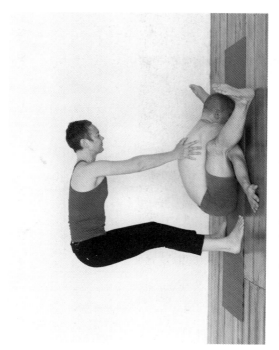

To set the foundation: Place the hands either side of the spine where the spine curves.

To adjust: Press directly down – very gently.

Supta Kurmasana

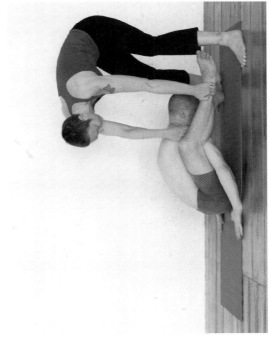

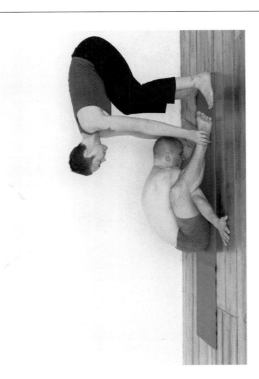

To adjust: First lift up the feet and bring them closer together. At the same time, bend the knees up.

The priority is to get the shoulders as far under the legs as comfortably possible – this will make binding much easier.

Ask the student to turn their palms up to the ceiling and stretch back (as if they were trying to touch the wall behind them).

As they stretch back, lift up their legs to create more space.

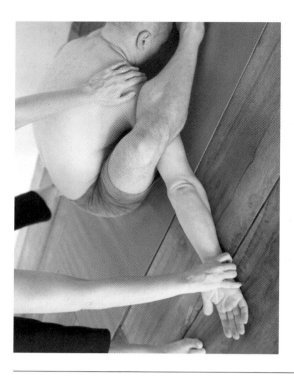

Next for the bind.

To set the foundation: Stand behind the student.

With one hand rotate the shoulder forwards and down.

With the other hand hold the wrist and draw the arm directly out to the side (it is important that the student completely relaxes at this point).

Then fold the arm across the back as high up as possible.

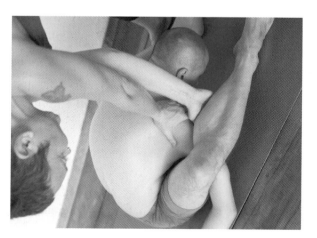

Then rotate the shoulder forwards and down and the calf muscle up (lateral rotation of lower leg) to tuck the shoulders under the legs.

Then hold the arms above the elbow and draw the hands together.

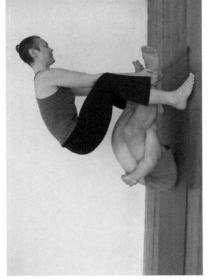

Final posture: Then step forwards so you are standing either side of their ankles.

Pick up the feet and bring them as close as comfortable – if possible, cross the right over the left.

Support most of their weight on your inner legs.

Notes: Be aware of your own posture, especially your back. If the hands cannot bind, give the student a towel to hold. When bringing the feet closer, make sure the shoulders don't hunch forwards, as the collarbones are vulnerable here.

If you are adjusting a student for the first time, explain to them what you are doing. Always make sure the student is relaxed – if they tense up or try to help you it just makes it harder for you and for them.

To set the foundation: Step forwards so you are standing either side of their knees.

Again, rotate the shoulders forwards and down and the calf muscle up.

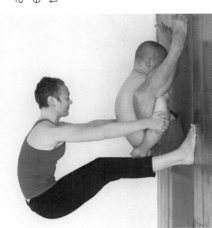

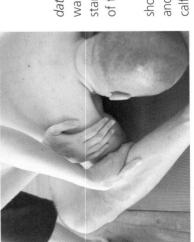

Garbha Pindasana

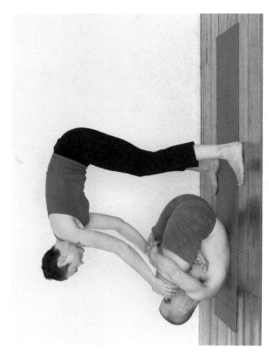

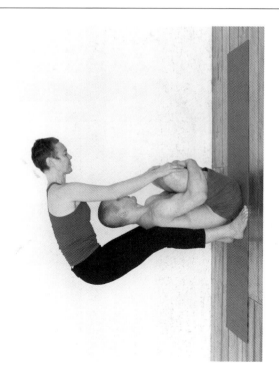

To set the foundation: Stand behind the student and use the inside of your lower legs either side of their spine for support.

To adjust: Take the student's knees and gently lift up and back.

To help rolling around: Hold the student's knees and rock them round.

Baddha Konasana

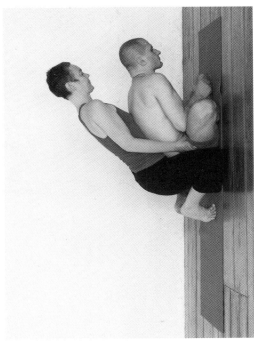

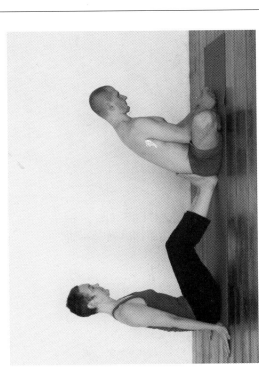

If the student is fairly upright in the posture try this version of the adjustment.

To set the foundation: Sitting behind the student, place your feet either side of the spine at the top of the hips.

To adjust: Gently push forwards and up.

If the student can go further forwards, try this.

To set the foundation: Place your hands mid-thigh and press directly down (if the hips are very stiff place your hands closer in towards the body and externally rotate the hips (draw them back and down).

To adjust: Keeping gentle pressure down on the legs, place your abdomen on the lower back. Ease the student gently forwards as they exhale.

Baddha Konasana B

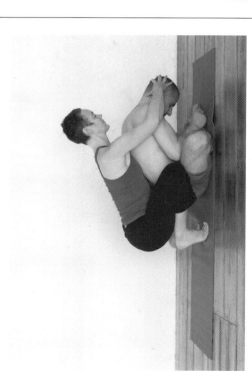

To set the foundation: Place your knees either side of their hips as close in towards the body as you can.

To adjust: Place your hands over their head with the thumbs pressing into the dents in the occipital bone. Place your abdomen on the student's back. Gently take them forwards and down.

Upavishta Konasana

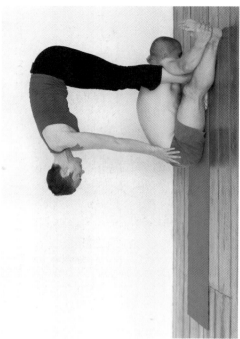

To set the foundation: Stand between the legs and arms with the back of your legs against the top of their arms.

To adjust: Use your hands to ground the sitting bones or the tops of the thighs back and down. Press back with the backs of your legs to create length through the spine.

Note: This adjustment can cause the shoulders to hunch a bit, but it is very effective at creating length in the spine.

Do not do this adjustment on people already very low down; it works best on people half way down.

Supta Padangushtasana

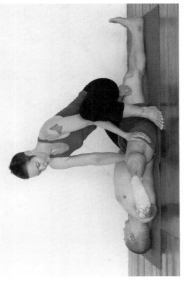

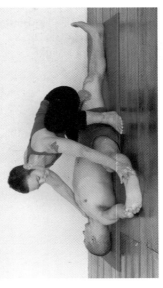

As they take their leg out to the side, encourage an outwards rotation in the leg (lateral rotation).

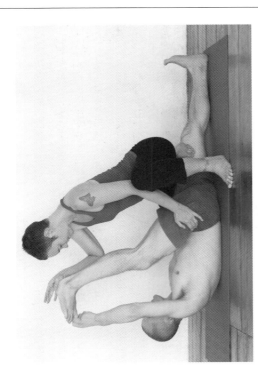

To set the foundation: Kneel so you can use your right knee to hold the left leg down towards the floor.

To adjust: Use your left hand to draw their right hip down and in towards the centre line. Use your right hand to ease the leg down.

Use your right hand to press down on either the shoulder or the left hip.

Use your left hand to ease the foot down towards the floor.

Urdhva Mukha Paschimattanasana

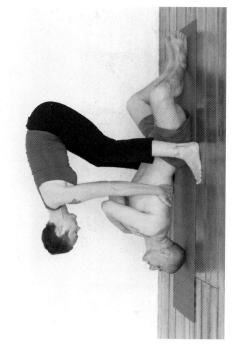

To set the foundation: Stand behind the student with the insides of your legs supporting either side of the spine.

To adjust: Cup their ankles with your hands and draw them up and back towards you.

Setu Bandhasana

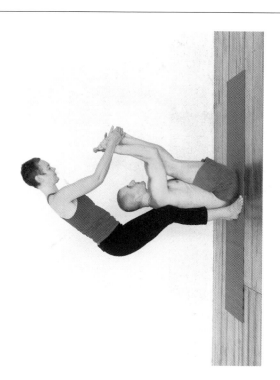

This adjustment is to give a bit of support and stability, not to take someone deeper.

To set the foundation: Stand with your feet either side of the student's hips. Place your hands under their body just below the shoulder blades.

FINISHING POSTURES

Urdhva Dhanurasana

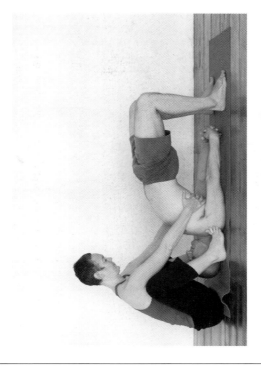

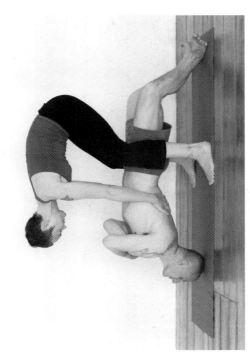

To adjust: Support them as they lift up. Once they are up, squeeze their hips with your legs.

Note: Watch your own posture and lower back.

Try this if the student is doing a half back-bend.

To set the foundation: Sit at the student's head and use your feet to ground the shoulders down.

To adjust: Place your hands just under the shoulder blades and lift them up and towards you.

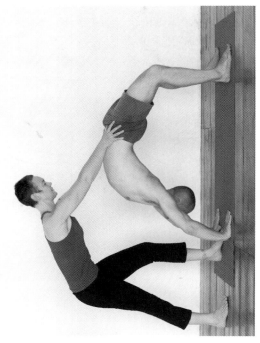

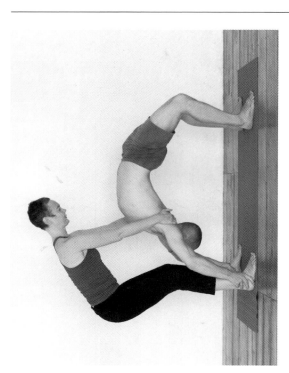

Use this if the student needs help lifting up (generally if the shoulders are tight or weak).

To set the foundation: Stand at the student's head with your feet hip-width apart. Let them hold your ankles.

To adjust: Hold either side of the shoulders and lift up and towards you.

Try the following adjustments if the student is comfortably in the posture.

To set the foundation: Stand at the student's head.

To adjust: Place your hands on their hips and ask them to press up into your hands. As they do so, give equal and opposite pressure back. This gives the student resistance to work against and enables them to lift up into the posture themselves.

SUGGESTED READING

Yoga: The Art of Adjusting by Brian Cooper (Harmony Publishing, 2010)

REFERENCES

1   Swami Niranjanananda Saraswati, *Prana, Pranayama, Prana Vidya* (Yoga Publications Trust, Bihar, 1994), p. 9

2   Coulter, David H, *Anatomy of Hatha Yoga: A Manual For Students, Teachers and Practitioners* (Body and Breath, Honesdale, 2001), p. 557

3   Ibid, p. 90

4   Saraswati, as above, p. 39

5   McCall, Timothy, *Yoga as Medicine: The yoga prescription for health and healing* (Bantam Books, New York, 2007), pp. 277–8, 392, 452–3, 471, 421, 367, 374

6   Ibid, p. 39

7   Saraswati, as above, p. 32

8   Coulter, p. 90 and Saraswati, as above, p. 38

9   McCall, pp 54 and Gore, Makarand M., *Anatomy and Physiology of Yogic Practices* (New Age Books, Delhi, 2005), pp. 27–9

10 Saraswati, as above, p. 192

11 McCall, p. 367

12 Ibid p. 183

13 Ibid pp. 40–41

14 Saraswati, as above, p. 40

15 Coulter, p. 557

16 Ibid, p. 557

17 Saraswati, as above, p. 39

18 Hinwood, Barry G., *A Textbook of Science for the Health Professionals* (Nelson Thornes, 1997), e-book

19 B.K.S. Iyengar, *Light on Pranayama: The Yogic Art of Breathing*, The Crossroad Publishing Company, New York 2010 p. 20 and Ray Long, *The Key Muscles of Yoga* (Bandha Yoga Publications, Canada, 2005) pp. 212–3

20 Gore, pp. 27–9

21 Iyengar, p. 26 and Maehle, Gregor, *Ashtanga Yoga; Practice and Philosophy* (Kaivalya Publications, Australia, 2006), p. 10

22 Sweeney, Matthew, *Yoga As It Is* (Australia, 2005), p. 14

23 Gore, Makarand M., *Anatomy and Physiology of Yogic Practices* (New Age Books, Delhi, 2005) p. 145 and Swami Baddhananda, *Moola Bandha: The Master Key* (Bihar School of Yoga, Bihar, 1978), p. 4

24 Baddhananda, p. 3

25 Ibid and Gore, p.p 142

26 Maehle, p. 12

27 Gore, p. 76 and p. 147

28 Gore, p. 149

29 Ibid p. 149

30 Ibid p. 149

31 Maehle, p. 75

32 Gore, p. 145

33 Ibid p. 145

34 Ibid p. 145

35 Ibid p. 145

36 Swami Satyananada Saraswati, *Asana Pranayama Mudra Bandha* (Bihar School of Yoga, India, 1969), p. 481

37 Gore, p. 176

38 Sweeney, p. 12

39 McCall, p. 41

40 Bates, W.H., *Better eyesight without glasses: retrain your eyes and rediscover 20/20 vision* (Hind Pocket Books, 2003), e-book

41 Cope, Stephen, *Yoga and the Quest for the True Self* (Bantam Books, 1999) p. 37

42 McCall, p. 49

43 Sri K. Pattabhi Jois, *Yoga Mala* (North Point Press, 1999), p. 6

44 Ibid p. 12

45 Saraswati, as above, p. 44

46 Schiffmann, Eric, *Yoga: the spirit and practice of moving into stillness* (Pockett Books, 1996) p. 64

47 Farhi, Donna, *Teaching yoga: exploring the teacher-student relationship* (Rodmell Press, 2006), e-book